MAGNETIC APPEAL

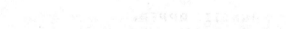

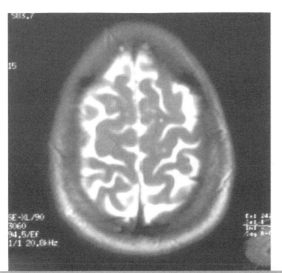

MAGNETIC APPEAL

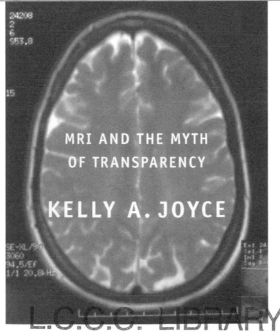

MRI AND THE MYTH
OF TRANSPARENCY

KELLY A. JOYCE

CORNELL UNIVERSITY PRESS
Ithaca and London

First published 2008 by Cornell University Press
First printing, Cornell Paperbacks, 2008

Printed in the United States of America

Library of Congress Cataloging-in-Publication Data

Joyce, Kelly A. (Kelly Ann), 1966–
    Magnetic appeal: MRI and the myth of transparency / Kelly A. Joyce.
        p.   cm.
    Includes bibliographical references and index.
    ISBN 978-0-8014-4489-0 (cloth : alk. paper)–
    ISBN 978-0-8014-7456-9 (pbk. : paper)
    1. Magnetic resonance imaging.   2. Magnetic resonance imaging–United States.   I. Title.
RC78.7.N83J69 2008
616.07'548–dc22   2007048070

Cornell University Press strives to use environmentally responsible suppliers and materials to the fullest extent possible in the publishing of its books. Such materials include vegetable-based, low-VOC inks and acid-free papers that are recycled, totally chlorine-free, or partly composed of nonwood fibers. For further information, visit our website at www.cornellpress.cornell.edu.

Cloth printing   10 9 8 7 6 5 4 3 2 1
Paperback printing   10 9 8 7 6 5 4 3 2 1

Contents

Acknowledgments

Many people contributed to this book. Of the many who shared their time and ideas, I want to highlight the following.

I thank the physicians, technologists, and scientists who discussed their professional training, work practices, and perspectives on medicine with me. Without their participation this book would not exist. I also thank the data specialists who helped me along the way. Researchers at the American College of Radiology, American Medical Association, American Society of Radiologic Technologists, Centers for Medicare and Medicaid Services, Food and Drug Administration, General Electric, Hitachi, Virginia Commonwealth University Medical Center, and Radiological Society of North America provided invaluable data for this book.

My investigations of medical imaging technologies began at Boston College. The faculty and students in the sociology department created an open-minded, vibrant intellectual milieu. I especially thank Jeanne Guillemin, Stephen Pfohl, Juliet Schor, Stefan Timmermans, and Diane Vaughan for their careful reading and constructive feedback on my writing and for their support over the years.

As the book evolved, I benefited from the contributions of the editors and staff at Cornell University Press. Peter Wissoker's subtle humor and helpful advice made the book writing process an enjoyable journey. I thank Ange Romeo-Hall for superb editing and Susan Barnett for exceptional marketing and publicity. I appreciate the anonymous reviewers' suggestions for the manuscript. Their insightful criticisms made *Magnetic Appeal* a stronger piece of analytical work.

Family and friends gave multiple forms of support for this project. Donna Joyce, Edward Scanlon, Shirley Scanlon, Mari Sullivan, Jim Sullivan, and Kate Sullivan provided writing havens and good company. Alice Joyce and Jack Joyce shared plant-, food-, and art-related adventures. Christy Burns, Jane Geaney, Elaine Marolla, and Shashwat Pandhi joined me for long urban hikes that helped clarify ideas and offered necessary respites.

The following people commented on components of this book. For this intellectual labor and gift, I thank Julia Garrett, Adria Goodson, David Hogge, Laura Holliday, Kimberly Mann, Elaine Marolla, Shashwat Pandhi, Celine Pascale, J. C. Poutsma, Timmons Roberts, Dee Royster, and Kate Slevin. I particularly thank Laura Mamo, T. L. Taylor, and Keith McGowan for dedicating time, energy, and good will to this project. Laura shared her friendship, professional wisdom, and careful editorial eye. T. L. listened to my ideas, offered sound advice, fielded emergency edits, and helped in the quest for clarity. Keith read every page of the manuscript at least once, talked through ideas, and offered enthusiasm and support throughout the writing process.

I thank the Schroeder Center for Healthcare Policy and the Office of the Provost at the College of William and Mary for financial support, and the Graduate School of Arts and Sciences of Boston College for a University Dissertation Fellowship. Parts of chapter 2 were published as "From Numbers to Pictures: The Development of Magnetic Resonance Imaging and the Visual Turn in Medicine," in *Science as Culture* (2006) 15(1): 1–22; and an early version of chapter 3 was published as "Appealing Images: Magnetic Resonance Imaging and the Construction of Authoritative Knowledge," in *Social Studies of Science* (2005) 35(3): 437–462.

I dedicate this book to my mother, Donna Joyce. I learned the value of steadfastness and style from her work ethic and keen imagination. Growing up reading her nursing books and magazines taught me to love and enjoy science. Listening to her stories about medicine helped me understand the human dimensions of health care.

MAGNETIC APPEAL

MRI as Cultural Icon

I n the June 10, 2004, episode of the popular soap opera *General Hospital,* a conversation between Emily and Nikolas about Nikolas's head injury reflects a common view of magnetic resonance imaging technology, also known as MRI or MR:[1]

NIKOLAS: The doctor said I should start with an MRI.
EMILY: Okay.
NIKOLAS: He said that that will determine if there's any damage to any specific area of my brain, but I—you know, I—I got to tell you, Emily, I—I don't know if I am ready to deal with the reality that the person I used to be is gone forever. I don't—
EMILY: But if there's the chance that your brain wasn't damaged.
NIKOLAS: Look, it's been months now, and I don't remember one thing.

---

[1] I use the acronym MRI to denote magnetic resonance imaging in this book. This is the label currently used by lay people and some medical personnel to discuss this technology. However, many radiologists, technologists, and medical imaging salespeople use the term MR instead of MRI. The use of MR allows manufacturers and medical professionals to distinguish between the different types of MRI examinations currently available. It promotes discussion of magnetic resonance angiography, for example, which are images of blood vessels, and magnetic resonance spectroscopy, which uses magnetic resonance technology to measure biochemicals such as choline in the body. Shortening MRI to MR opens up the space for acronyms such as MRA or MRS. The term MR may replace the phrase MRI in the popular imagination as these procedures become more common.

EMILY: Okay . . . If the MRI shows permanent damage and you may
never remember your past, then you could let go and move on and
focus on the present, on the future, create a new life for yourself
however you choose to do it.

NIKOLAS: I don't know, okay? I don't know.

EMILY: But if the scan shows that you could recapture who you used to
be, you'd be able to fill in the blanks. You could get answers to all
of your questions. All right, you'd feel complete and whole. How
can you possibly pass up that chance?

In this dialogue, MRI, a technology used to create anatomical pictures, is
deemed a crucial component of medical practice. It is what the doctor
"starts with" and is presented as the main technology used in diagnostic
work. Other intriguing aspects of this dialogue are the assumptions that
MRI examinations can reveal the truth about one's physical condition,
produce a definitive medical diagnosis, and reveal one's identity. From the
MRI scan, Nikolas may be able to "recapture who he used to be" or, if he
needs to, "create a new life." Based on these claims, refusing an examination is equivalent to forgoing knowledge about both one's body and one's
self. And as Emily understandably concludes, "How can you possibly pass
up that chance?"

The implication in the dialogue that MRI is both a starting point of
medical treatment and an infallible diagnostic instrument is not unusual.
From exhibits at Disney's Epcot and cartoons in the *New Yorker* magazine
to Patricia Cornwell's crime novel *Predator*, MRI is commonly framed as a
cutting-edge technique that is crucial to contemporary medical practice
and research. The technology and its benefits are often referred to in
popular culture, science exhibits, news stories, and policy debates to the
point that MRI can be considered a *cultural icon*—a sacred object on
which revolve questions about personal health, identity, and life's many
dilemmas.

Magnetic Appeal examines the cultural, political, and economic factors
that contribute to the making of MRI as a cultural icon. By tracing the narratives used in the public sphere, this book describes how MRI is transformed into a technology of truth that not only symbolizes quality health
care but also has the power to reveal facts about one's medical condition.
The book begins with the scientists who created MRI and follows the technology into clinical medicine. Fieldwork at imaging units and radiology
conferences and interviews with physicians and technologists provide an
understanding of MRI *in practice*. By accompanying the actors who create
and use anatomical images, this book shows how cultural ideas about the

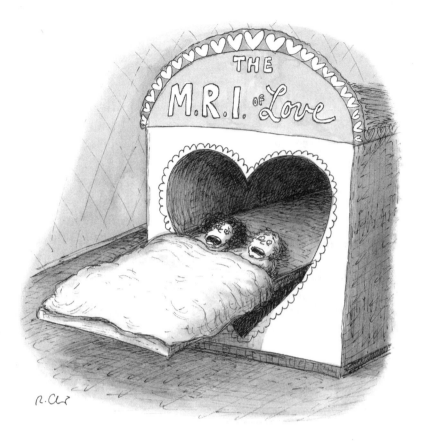

"The M.R.I. of Love," by Roz Chast. *Source*: The *New Yorker* Collection 2003, Roz Chast from cartoonbank.com. All Rights Reserved.

technology and the work conditions of diagnostic health care professionals make MRI into what sociologists Adele Clarke and Joan Fujimura (1992) call the "right tool for the job" even though it cannot always deliver the certainty promised on television or in the news media.

What cultural beliefs and economic factors enabled MRI to become a technology of truth? How do medical professionals create, use, and make sense of anatomical images in their work? How does a medical professional's decision to order an MRI examination relate to broader trends in medicine such as the fear of litigation, the pressure to produce more revenue, the push to see more patients in a given time period, and the effort to establish marketing relationships between manufacturers and physicians? Finally, what is the relationship between the use and even the invention of MRI and the sociotechnical turn toward visualization? In what

way does the escalating use of MRI and the presumption of truth attributed to the anatomical images it creates contribute to the deepening faith
people place in that very same technology?

Magnetic Appeal answers these questions and shows how MRI
technology—its creation, use, and meanings—brings together cultural
ideas about vision and technology, professional expertise and knowledge,
and the economic and institutional dimensions of medicine. Using sociological theories of science and technology, fieldwork observations, and in-
depth interviews with medical professionals and scientists, this book shows
how the desire for and use of MRI technology cannot be understood outside of cultural and institutional contexts.

Technology and Biomedicine

MRI technology was introduced to clinical practice in the 1980s. It was initially used to make pictures of the brain, the spine, and the area around
the joints. Today, MRI technology is used to visualize the heart, breasts,
liver, arteries, and other soft tissues in the body. Physicians, chiropractors,
nurse practitioners, and other licensed medical professionals primarily
order scans as a diagnostic tool. These MRI examinations, like many other
medical tests, are conducted outside the offices of referring medical professionals. Medical practitioners then evaluate the examination results in
relation to other clinical findings to formulate diagnoses for patients.

More recently, MRI has moved from diagnostic tool to treatment intervention. For example, MRI-guided surgery has traveled from the
fringes of biomedicine to accepted practice (Carrino and Jolesz 2005).
In such cases, surgeons work with both real-time images and the body
when they operate on a patient. In an iterative process, surgeons monitor
changes in pictorial information and use this information to guide surgical interventions.

MRI technology is not reserved just for people. For many years, veterinarians have ordered scans for diagnostic purposes for their
patients—cats, dogs, and other animals—at teaching hospitals. They also
occasionally prescribed scans for animals that were then conducted at
human imaging facilities. Today, however, machines are designed with
animals' bodies in mind, and enterprising veterinarians and companies
are opening independent imaging centers (Krasner 2004; Strunksy
2002). For example, the Veterinary MRI and Radiotherapy Center in
New Jersey—the first private center in the United States—opened its
doors in 2002, and the Iams company, a division of Proctor and Gamble

and a producer of pet food, finances the construction of pet imaging centers nationwide.[2]

Not everyone has access to MRI examinations. Most people cannot afford nor are willing to pay for scans of their pets. More important, some people cannot afford the examinations for themselves. High copayments or lack of health insurance makes MRI scans, which generally range in price from $400 to $1000, too costly for many people. Moreover, race, gender, and geographic location (e.g., urban versus rural) may influence whether a person gets referred for an examination. After examining the behavior of 200 practitioners and 1580 patients, for instance, Carey and Garrett (1996) found that white people were more likely to receive an MRI than black people. While one study cannot be generalized, research on other technologies demonstrates how factors such as class, gender, race, and location influence patient access to medical procedures (see, e.g., Ford, Newman, and Deosaransing 2000; Fox and Swazey 1992; IOM 2002; Lillie, Blanton, Rushing, and Ruiz 2002; Roth 1997; Schulmenn et al. 1999). More research needs to be conducted to determine the relationship between social, geographic, and economic factors and MRI use.

Despite its high cost and unequal access, MRI use continues to grow. Each year the number of scans conducted on human beings increases, due in part to new applications of the technology (Bell 2004; Information Means Value [IMV] 2005). What was once primarily a tool for visualizing the brain and muscles around the spine and joints has moved far beyond these initial uses. Approximately 26.6 million MRI examinations were performed on people in the United States in 2006, and that number is expected to rise (IMV 2007). There are no figures available for the number of examinations conducted on animals, but the purchase and use of equipment by veterinarians demonstrate its increasing presence in providing health care for animals.

One explanation for the MRI boom draws on the "it is the best technology" line of reasoning. What this argument suggests is that we use the technology because it adds to diagnostic accuracy and better treatment outcomes for patients. Yet studies that compare MRI to other diagnostic techniques create a much more complex picture of how its use contributes to diagnostic work.[3] For example, published studies that examine

---

[2] The Veterinary MRI and Radiology Center's website is: http://www.vetmrirt.com/.

[3] Research on other imaging techniques such as computed tomography (CT) or x-ray creates a complex view of the contributions of imaging technology to the production of health (see, e.g., Haydel et al. 2000; Hoffman et al. 2000; Miller et al. 2002; Olsen and Gotzsche 2000). While imaging use adds to diagnostic confidence in specific cases, it does not necessarily improve the quality of diagnostic work or health outcomes for patients in all of the situations in which it is currently used.

the diagnosis of knee and shoulder muscle disorders show that while an MRI examination contributes valuable information in particular cases (Rose and Gold 1996), it does not produce the most valuable or cost-effective information in the diagnosis of many common shoulder and knee muscle problems (Gelb et al. 1996; Liu et al. 1996). In these cases, the combination of patient histories and physical exam techniques often provide more accurate information about a patient's condition than the knowledge produced through MRI. These studies show that, at best, the MRI examination simply replicates the information gained from a detailed history and a physical exam.

MRI is clearly important to health care work, but its status as an icon and the way its use has rapidly expanded cannot be understood solely through the "we use it because it is the best" explanation. While efficacy and utility can contribute to a technology's use, cultural ideas and values, policies, institutional practices, and economic relations all contribute to its symbolic meanings and applications. The diffusion and use of any technology is a social and cultural process that varies by technique, nation, and time period (Bijker 1995; Bradsher 2002; Cowan 1983; Oudshoorn 2003). This book examines the widespread use and generally positive framing of MRI technology in the United States. At the crossroads of sociology and science and technology studies (STS), *Magnetic Appeal* highlights the social, material, cultural, and economic factors that transform MRI technology into a desirable knowledge-producing technique.

The Growth of Visualization Technologies

A central argument of this book is that the development of MRI technology and our desire to use it must be understood in relation to the broader sociotechnical turn toward visualization. From family pictures and personal videos to the mass media of television, movies, and newspapers, we are inclined to represent life in picture form and to perceive the stories pictures present as meaningful representations of events, social relations, and people. Visualization provides us with a powerful way of seeing ourselves, our worlds, and our social relations from new and different perspectives. Biomedical practices are part of this sociotechnical turn: They simultaneously contribute to and are shaped by the proliferation of the ways in which we represent ourselves and our world visually. Moreover, cultural ideologies that link sight and knowledge contribute to how we find meaning in pictures of the body.

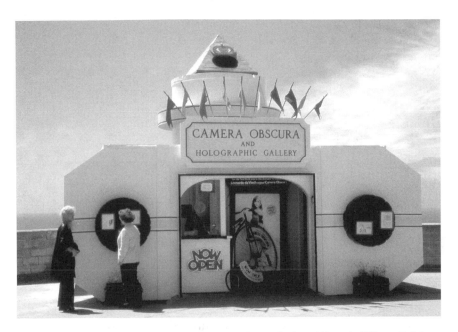

The Giant Camera, San Francisco, California. *Source*: Jack and Beverly Wilgus, Bright Bytes Studio.

Throughout the 1800s and early 1900s, the use of pictorial images proliferated in private and public spaces in the United States (Clarke 2004; Mirzoeff 1998; Sturken and Cartwright 2001). Camera obscura rooms, stereoscopes, photographs, and film cameras all provided ways to visualize life. For example, camera obscura rooms were popular attractions along the East and West coasts, and at waterfalls and other scenic spots (Wilgus and Wilgus 2006). Each room, through the use of a small hole in the wall, projected the outside scene onto a wall in the darkened interior. People paid money to see the projected scene, and they appreciated the camera obscura technique of picture making. Photographic and moving picture cameras were patented during the late 1800s, providing more techniques for visualizing life (Barger and White 2000; Crary 1990; Jenkins 1975). Tied to tourism, consumerism, and journalism, such technologies presented stories, scenes, and human relations as pictures.

Throughout the early and mid-twentieth century, people, regardless of their political views, increasingly used documentary photographs and films to communicate information about social worlds and experiences. Newspapers, films, and television programs used images to continue to uncritically depict dimensions of social life. At the same time, images were used to challenge inequalities and oppressions. For example, photographs and films provided evidence of the Holocaust, the brutality of the police during civil rights protests, and the harm caused by the Vietnam War on the Vietnamese people (Horstein and Jacobowitz 2002; Willis 2005). Images of these events filled television screens and newspapers and became a powerful way to convey knowledge about significant social events. Such practices helped shore up the idea that pictures reveal the truth about life and death.

The trend toward visualization intensified in the 1980s and 1990s as video cameras and recorders, photocopying machines, cable television, and computer visualization technologies became more available. No longer used just to tell public space stories or provide tourist attractions, machines such as cameras and computers were designed for personal use at home, at work, or while traveling. From cameras and copiers to camcorders and picture-producing cell phones, visualization devices enable us to represent ourselves and our relations to others through technologically produced images.

Mechanically reproduced sound (e.g., dialogues, soundtracks, and sound effects) can work with visual information to create and convey meaning. However, the senses of touch, smell, and taste have not experienced nearly the same degree of mechanical transformation as sight and sound (Corbin 1986, 1998; Jay 1994). Although art forms such as odorama cinema bring smell to visual representations, such endeavors are anomalies in a milieu that privileges the visual.

The move toward visualization has a long history in medicine—one that is tied to an increasing emphasis on surveillance. Scholars of science, technology, and medicine provide critical analyses of medicine's visual culture and examine the deployment of cameras and other visualizing devices in health care and research (see, e.g., Beaulieu 2000; Cartwright 1995; Dumit 2004; Hartouni 1997; Treichler, Cartwright, and Penley 1998; Waldby 2000). Michel Foucault locates the emergence of the insistence on visuality, or what he calls the "clinical gaze," in eighteenth-century Europe.

> [This period is one in which] illness, counter-nature, death, in short, the whole dark underside of disease came to light, at the same time illuminating and eliminating itself like night, in the deep, visible, solid, enclosed, but accessible space of the human body. What was fundamentally invisible is suddenly offered to the brightness of the gaze, in a movement of appearance so simple, so immediate that it seems to be the natural consequence of a more highly developed experience. (Foucault 1975, 195)

Assigning advantage to a way of knowing that centers on "a world of constant visibility," the clinical gaze insists on making the interior body exterior (Foucault 1975, x). The gaze normalizes the manipulation of the inner body, allowing the customization of bodies at the cellular and genetic level (Clarke 1995; Clarke et al. 2003; Squier 2004). From this era on, medical knowledge and practice insist on rendering inner spaces and processes seemingly transparent. One way medical professionals did this was to develop and employ medical imaging technologies.

Throughout the early twentieth century, the ability to produce anatomical images mechanically was limited. The primary imaging technique for making pictures of the inner body was x-ray technology (Blume 1992; Kevles 1997).[4] X-ray technologies were wildly popular and captured everyone's imagination, scientists and the average citizen alike. Health care professionals relied almost exclusively on x-rays to make pictures of the internal body since other imaging technologies either were not readily available or did not exist. At the same time, x-ray machines were used in shoe stores to make pictures of the bones in the foot because salespeople claimed its use enabled better fittings. Other people, due to curiosity, paid out of pocket to have parts of their body x-rayed (Kevles 1997, 58). Concern about the harmful effects of radiation and the increasing professional authority of physicians eventually limited the use of x-ray in consumer sites. By the 1950s, x-ray machines disappeared from shoe stores and other consumer-oriented businesses, leaving the imaging device under the primary control of medical professionals (Duffin and Hayter 2000).

The availability and range of medical imaging technologies changed radically during the second half of the twentieth century. As part of a broader social investment in science and technology after World War II, researchers explored ways to extend and transform existing scientific techniques such as sonar, x-ray, radioactive tracers, and nuclear magnetic resonance to produce knowledge about the internal body and health (Blume 1992; Kevles 1997; Wobarst 1999). This research culminated in imaging technologies such as ultrasound, computed tomography (CT), and magnetic resonance imaging, which were introduced to hospitals and clinical practice in the 1970s and 1980s. As with x-ray, these newer visualization technologies also captured the public's imagination. By the 2000s, companies used anatomical pictures as logos, and consumers who could afford

[4] For social and cultural histories of particular technologies, see Golan (1998) and Pasveer (1989) for x-ray, Yoxen (1987) for ultrasound, and Dumit (2004) for positron emission tomography (PET).

the expense purchased scans of their inner bodies at shopping malls or at private businesses (Barnard 2000; Garza 2005).

MRI and the Power of the Visual

Computer-based medical imaging technologies are integral to contemporary epistemologies of the body. That is, how we know and understand the body is shaped through cultural conventions and practices. Today, these technologies include x-ray, ultrasound, CT, MRI, positron emission tomography (PET), and single photon emission computed tomography (SPECT). Medical professionals refer to them as an imaging armamentarium, and their hold on the imagination has intensified over the years as the public's perception of their capabilities has grown. The growth in medical visualization technologies contributes to the proliferation of images in daily life as biomedical practitioners create and circulate visual products for our consumption. Embraced by medical professionals, journalists, artists, and consumers, computer-based imaging technologies have become part of our popular culture.

Visualization supports the production and use of medical imaging in two primary ways. First, the use of images in all areas of social life and the relative ease with which they are created provide the technological innovation needed to make medical imaging a routine practice. Imaging techniques are hybrid technologies. Each relies on innovations in computer processing and information technologies to produce and display pictures in a timely fashion. Without such innovations, the development and integration of MRI, CT, and ultrasound into medical care would have been impossible.

Second, the meaning ascribed to a photograph contributes to making an anatomical image desirable. Cultural narratives commonly attribute truth to photographic images, and that truth is ascribed to the thing or person represented in the image (Sturken and Cartwright 2001; Berger 1973; Sontag 1990). Although the view exists that images are posed and constructed, the idea that pictures represent a transparent window of the world remains strong (van Dijck 2005). In a symbolic economy that equates photographic pictures with the person or object represented, medical images appear to offer the possibility of accessing the inner body without mediation to discover truth. When people are sick or in pain, such access is perceived as necessary since it is believed to provide the correct diagnosis needed to alleviate suffering.

The claim of truth is staked partially on the terrain of the visual: For something to be true, it must be seen. This point is illustrated when patients with mental illness and their families support brain imaging as a way to prove to skeptical scientists and policy makers that disease exists and research funding is needed (Dumit 2000). Culture, interest groups, and power determine whether knowledge is perceived as trustworthy, and what counts as evidence varies across time and place. Numbers (Porter 1995), clinical trials (Timmermans and Berg 2003), genetics, and images are all publicly recognized as potentially trustworthy sources of information. To fight for truth and legitimacy is often to fight within these arenas.

MRI in particular benefits from the certainty ascribed to images. Within the panoply of visualization technologies, MRI is given high status. Although each technology has situations in which it is the most appropriate and valuable, MRI is considered the gold standard of medical imaging techniques by both medical professionals and the general public. It symbolizes top-of-the-line health care and is one of the most expensive imaging machines available. Its public perception as the gold standard spills onto the image itself. If pictures in general provide an unmediated window into the body, then MRI as a high-status machine that generates an entire series of pictures must produce even more accurate and certain knowledge.

How MRI Works

Reflecting the importance of visualization in contemporary life, technical and human interventions transform the original quantitative data obtained by CT, MRI, ultrasound, and PET into anatomical images without the use of a camera lens (Cartwright and Goldfarb 1992). Ultrasound, for example, uses transmitters to produce high-frequency sound waves that are reflected by soft tissue in the body. The transducer, a component of the technology, detects the strength and time of the resulting echoes (Wobarst 1999, 132), and these values are transformed via computer programs into ultrasound images. Like ultrasound, MRI exemplifies the trend of making anatomical pictures without a camera lens. Despite being a picture-producing machine, MRI is initially used to make numerical measurements of the activity of hydrogen atoms in the body. Each technique—ultrasound, MRI, CT, and PET—utilizes a different aspect of scientific knowledge to produce images of the inner body. Humans then work with these hybrid technologies to manufacture information about a patient's body in visual form.

For MRI, there are two main machine designs available. The first, called an open MRI machine, allows patients to have open spaces on either side of their body while in the machine. The second, referred to as a closed

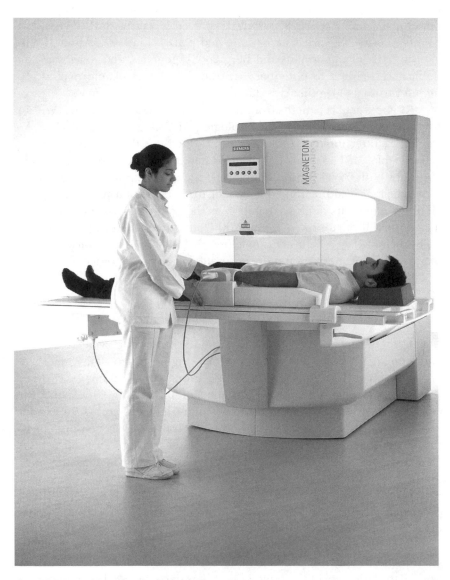

Open MRI machine. *Source*: Siemens Press Pictures.

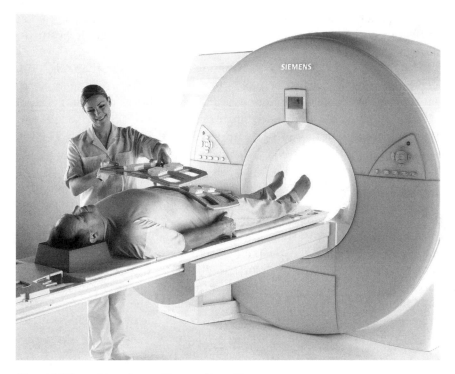

Closed MRI machine. *Source*: Siemens Press Pictures.

MRI machine, requires patients to be in a closed tunnel or tube during the scan. Although the final output of each examination is a series of anatomical pictures, each picture represents a complex series of steps, all of which are needed to produce the final image.

Each machine contains a main magnet—usually a superconducting magnet—that creates a generally uniform and constant magnetic field around the machine. To begin an examination, the MRI technologist directs the patient into the machine, and thus into this field. This placement causes the nuclei of the patient's hydrogen atoms, which are part of the water in and around a person's cells, to align with the magnetic field. In other words, it causes the nuclei to act like tiny compass needles that point in the direction produced by the external magnetic field. The technologist then directs the machine to beam pulses of radio frequency waves at the patient's body. The hydrogen nuclei absorb these energy waves, which causes them to flip over and point in the opposite direction. The absorption of energy also causes the nuclei to rotate "in phase" or together. Wire coils near the patient's body measure the new positions of the hydrogen nuclei, and these signals are recorded and stored in a computer. Once this information is recorded in the computer, the technologist turns off the radio frequency waves.

Computer programs, using information obtained from the coils, also record the time it takes for the nuclei to release the absorbed energy and return to their original alignment with the external magnetic field. These relaxation times are numbers. Each numerical value is then coded and transformed via computer software into a component of an image. The re-configured numerical measurements are compiled to create an anatomi-cal picture of the inner body. Each MRI scan thus represents a series of translations. The body is transformed into an array of numerical measure-ments that are then coded into images. The images are then interpreted by a physician, who is usually a radiologist, in a written report.

One outgrowth of MRI is the tendency to represent the body as multiple images. Moving beyond the one-picture output associated with x-ray exami-nations, post-1950s technologies such as ultrasound, CT, PET, and MRI pro-duce a series of pictures of the inner body from different perspectives. This multiplicity of images has the effect of enhancing the credibility of MRI technology and the visual knowledge produced. If one picture is believed to reveal the body and the truth it holds, then numerous images create a trans-parency surplus—one that overflows with the promise of unmediated ac-cess to the inner body. This promise—reinforced by medical terminology that labels each picture a "slice" of the body—reinforces the notion that anatomical pictures reveal the truth about bodies. And, in a reciprocal fash-ion, the fact that we believe that these images reveal truth contributes to a broader cultural perception that a connection exists between photographs and unmediated knowledge.

Users Matter: The Work Practices of Physicians and Technologists

The human actors who make and use MRI examinations in clinical prac-tice are the focus of this book. As science and technology studies (STS) scholars Nelly Oudshoorn and Trevor Pinch (2003, ix) note, "Users are everywhere gaining prominence."[5] Within STS and medical sociology, there has been a concerted effort to study the people who use techno-science (see, e.g., Cowan 1987; Pinch and Bijker 1984; Mamo 2007; Moore 1997). Users, who are predominantly framed as patients or consumers,

[5] The word "users" is also used in industry. In the business of information technology, the term *users* describes individuals who use a particular website, search engine, or program.

provide insight in the interpretations and uses of a technology. Technologies do not have intrinsic meanings or purposes that guide their use. Instead, social actors articulate their meanings and uses within particular situations and contexts (Clarke and Fujimura 1992, 27).

In this book, I broaden the definition of "users" beyond the lay public to include the professionals who create, interpret, and use MRI scans. Using fieldwork at three imaging sites and MRI-related conferences and in-depth interviews with forty-eight medical professionals, I focus on how radiologists, referring physicians, and technologists use and make sense of anatomical scans in clinical practice. I illustrate that the manner in which these professionals practice medicine reflects cultural, institutional, economic, and professional priorities, and these priorities in turn affect how MRI is used in practice.

Focusing on medical professionals shows how physicians and technologists are influenced by and contribute to culture. *Culture* refers to language, values, conventions, material objects, and identities; it comprises the symbolic and material worlds of a particular society (Oudshoorn 2003; Casper 1998, 16–17). A major argument of STS is that scientific work and the production of medical knowledge are cultural practices. As such, they are shaped by broader values, representational practices, and ideas (Lock 2002; Martin 1985, 1995). Analysis of the professionals who produce, interpret, and use MRI in clinical medicine illuminates one dimension of the science/culture tangle—the reciprocal relations that exist between scientists' ideas and actions and the emphasis on and meanings attributed to the visual.

The physicians and technologists I interviewed are understood as social actors whose language and views are not only shaped by but also contribute to cultural ideas about sight, machines, and knowledge. They often exemplify the ways in which the technologically produced visual is privileged as a powerful truth-telling medium. Socialized in a cultural milieu that connects evidence to the visual, clinical medical workers describe anatomical images in ways that emphasize their ability to render the body transparent. Their use of such narratives is not neutral. The views of these workers carry the weightiness of science, thus reinforcing the use of such narratives in other realms such as the media and popular culture.

By attending to the work practices of physicians and technologists, this book demonstrates three broader transformations in U.S. medicine. First, accompanying physicians and technologists in their daily activities demonstrates how medical workers—much like other workers—are under pressure to increase productivity: Volume and revenue drive work on the medical shop floor. All medical professionals, from referring practitioners to technologists to radiologists, are required to process patients and information faster. The emphasis on speed results in less time available for the evaluation of diagnostic information, shorter patient visits, and the steady progression of people through diagnostic tests.

Second, analysis of health care work illuminates how perceptions of litigation shape the contours of medical practice. Physicians are acutely aware of the specter of litigation and take steps to avoid possible lawsuits. These steps can include explaining risks and complications in detail to patients and ordering more diagnostic procedures such as MRI examinations (Klingman, Localio, and Sugarman 1996; Jacobson and Rosenquist 1996; Kachalia, Choudhry, and Studdert 2005). The heightened awareness of litigation has even led to the coining of phrases such as "cover your ass" medicine to describe the actions taken by practitioners to protect themselves.

Third, an observation of medical professionals demonstrates how hierarchies on the shop floor affect social interaction between workers in imaging units. The existence and effects of inequalities among nurses, doctors, and other health care workers has been well documented (Copnell et al. 2004; Davies 2003; Gordon 2005; Rosenstein 2002). In the case of MRI, technologists have less power and status than physicians and nurses, and an awareness of hierarchy weighs upon social and professional interactions among each group. Even when individuals try to view and treat colleagues as equals, professional status and alliances trump efforts to be egalitarian when time is short and frustrations fly; this, in turn, affects patient care. For example, professional hierarchies can make it harder for technologists to enforce safety precautions (e.g., keeping metal out of the exam room) among doctors and nurses, which can injure patients as well as health care professionals. The magnetic field produced by the MRI machine transforms metal objects into potentially dangerous projectiles that can harm any individual near the machine.

Biomedicine, Inc.

The actions of medical workers and beliefs about MRI cannot be understood without an in-depth analysis of economic relations and arrangements. While hospitals, medical professionals, and popular culture are vital in shaping the popular perception of the uses and capabilities of MRI, they are not alone. Companies such as General Electric, Siemens, and Hitachi—the main producers of imaging machines—play a fundamental role in shaping beliefs about MRI. *Magnetic Appeal* examines corporate practices to demonstrate how the desire for and use of MRI technology are shaped by both direct and indirect advertising to physicians, administrators, and patients, as well as the pursuit of corporate profits.

The connections among pharmaceutical industries, medical practice, and direct-to-consumer advertising have received significant attention (Abramson 2005; Angell 2004; Fishman 2004; Loe 2004; Sismondo 2004). Yet the relationships among imaging machine and parts manufacturers, clinicians, and patients have not been studied to the same extent. Examining these relationships adds to our understanding of the varied economic interactions that structure biomedical practice. For example, indirect advertising to patients is central to this realm of biomedicine. Unlike the pharmaceutical industry which relies on direct advertising to patients as well as clinicians, medical imaging companies rely on more subtle forms of promotion. The popular television show *House,* for example, exemplifies this practice through its regular inclusion of MRI machines in episodes. Representing a form of product placement familiar for objects such as computers and food items in cinema and television shows, General Electric Healthcare—a major producer of MRI machines—is a show sponsor.

How corporate relations structure the use of MRI is not addressed in the literature on medical imaging technologies. Previous literature assesses the popular meanings attributed to pictures of the inner body (Beaulieu 2000; Cartwright 1995, 1998; Hartouni 1997; Stabile 1992; Waldby 2000). For example, Lisa Cartwright (1998) shows how hegemonic ideas about family and gender were used to describe the male and female bodies pictured in the Visible Human Project. The project, funded by the National Library of Medicine, dissected and scanned two people who donated their bodies to science into thousands of images. Illustrating how heteronormative ideas structure scientific knowledge, some researchers described the bodies as "the Visible Couple" or a "digital Adam and Eve" even though the subjects did not know each other in life (Cartwright 1998, 29).[6] Scholars have also investigated how research scientists use and make sense of medical scans in laboratories (Beaulieu 2002; Dumit 2004; Prasad 2005a, 2005b). *Magnetic Appeal* contributes to the literature by extending the analytical field to include corporate relations and by focusing on clinical medicine. Addressing these topics pushes us to think about the connections between economics, cultural ideas, and the clinical uses of MRI technology.

---

[6] Heteronormativity highlights how heterosexuality is privileged in institutional practices, policies, and social relations (Ingraham 1994; Warner 1991). For example, birth certificates and adoption papers assume couples are heterosexual when they ask for the mother and father's names instead of using gender neutral terminology such as "parents."

The development of MRI technology highlights and solidifies interactions among individuals, organizations, the material world, and symbolic environments. Rejecting causal explanations, I trace the flows and linkages among medical professionals, popular ideas about MRI technology, and economic relationships to better understand how MRI is used in clinical practice. What we know today as MRI cannot be understood without examining the technology itself, the motivations and actions of actors, and the institutional and economic practices that influence how and when the technology is used and seen. Indeed, biomedical technologies are social, historical, and contingent artifacts. Due to ever-changing contexts and players, they are always open to cultural and technological reconfigurations and reconstructions.

Enter the Social Scientist: Researching MRI

My analysis of MRI draws on seven years of in-depth research that includes interviews, content analysis, fieldwork, and targeted literature reviews—all of which allowed me to understand different perspectives of the history and contemporary world of MRI. The material gained from this multi-method approach provides the basis for my analysis of this technology. To research the uses and perceptions of this technology, I developed an inclusive methodological approach that integrated fieldwork at hospitals and radiology conferences, in-depth interviews with physicians and technologists, content analysis of popular culture texts, and targeted literature reviews. This methodological tactic, which is detailed in the appendix, allowed me to investigate different ways of understanding MRI technology and to produce the complex view of medical imaging presented in this book.

For insight into the historical development of the technology, I conducted in-depth interviews with four researchers who contributed to the technology's invention and conducted archival research: Larry Crooks, Raymond Damadian, Paul Lauterbur, and John Mallard. Each worked at a different research site and provided insight into the context and decisions that shaped early MRI research. To understand the scientific innovations, political pressures, social actors, and social networks involved in the development of MRI technology, I also analyzed scientific papers and patents related to MRI, newspaper articles published during the 1970s and 1980s, and secondary historical accounts. From this research, I discovered that a sustained discussion of the cultural contexts in which MRI was created was often missing from standard histories.

To understand the symbolic meaning of MRI in the public realm, I analyzed the content of magazines, television shows, newspaper articles, popular science books, and exhibits. Coding the content of these sources clarified the recurring narratives used to describe the technology.

The fieldwork component of my research occurred at five MRI-related conferences and three different imaging units. I also interviewed referring physicians, radiologists, and technologists affiliated with the imaging units I observed. The fieldwork and in-depth interviews provided important information about the subjective meanings attached to this technology by those who use it. Fieldwork allowed me to observe how medical professionals discuss MRI. Listening to the discussions, asides, and jokes made by patients, technologists, and physicians provided insight into how these individuals made sense of the technology and their work practices. Fieldwork also allowed me to observe the interactions among technologists, physicians, and patients, including how power and inequality influenced social relations.

The perspectives gained by the interviews and fieldwork were complemented by a review of medical literature. I used the National Library of Medicine's electronic search engine PubMed/MEDLINE to investigate the types of studies that have been conducted about MRI use. I also reviewed print issues of *Radiology*, the *Journal of Magnetic Resonance Imaging*, and other MRI-related medical journals to better understand biomedical views of the technology. This focused literature review deepened my understanding and analysis of biomedical debates about what counts as scientific evidence, and allowed me to investigate the relations between accepted definitions of evidence and MRI use.

Overview of the Book

Each chapter of *Magnetic Appeal* offers a different glimpse of how local and national cultures, institutional practices, and social relationships shape our understanding and use of MRI. Although integral to the larger analysis, each chapter can also be read on its own as a series of what Donna Haraway (1997, 273) refers to as "diffractions" about MRI. Diffractions, as described by Haraway, evoke both the process and the effect of critical social investigation. This metaphor calls attention to how the act of examination itself is socially situated and subjective, and it also suggests how sociological analysis can spark meaningful dialogues and interventions. As diffractions, each chapter looks at an aspect of MRI, potentially generating conversations and actions related to health care that reverberate in unimagined yet consequential ways.

Chapter 2, "Painting by Numbers: The Development of Magnetic Resonance Imaging and the Visual Turn in Medicine," provides an institutional and cultural history of the development of MRI. Drawing on my interviews with the inventors of the technology and on secondary historical accounts, this chapter shows how the current practice of representing MRI data as gray scale images represents complex negotiations among research scientists, radiologists, and the public. This discussion illustrates how there is nothing natural or inevitable about the current form of MRI scans or the design of the technology itself. Instead, the invention of MRI is embedded in social relations and networks. As part of this analysis, the decision to turn the numerical data obtained by this technology into anatomical pictures is also examined. This decision anticipates the discussion of anatomical images and visuality that is central to the focus of this book.

Chapter 3, "Seeing Is Believing: The Transformation of MRI Examinations into Authoritative Knowledge," explores why MRI scans are compelling. Using data culled from fieldwork, interviews, and content analysis of media sources, this chapter illustrates how both media and medical narratives often suggest MRI examinations provide neutral knowledge that is equivalent to the physical body. Such narratives help create the idea that anatomical images reveal the truth about the body's interior and shore up the technology's desirability. This chapter also examines the production and interpretation processes that inscribe MRI exams. Comparing medical professionals' knowledge about their work practices with common narratives illustrates that transparency stories do not address how human decisions and values affect image content. By tracing the political effects of different views of MRI examinations, I assert that popular perceptions that equate the image with neutral knowledge make it harder to understand how health care policies, the desire to create revenue, and time constraints shape image quality.

To further analyze the social dimensions of MRI exams, chapter 4, "The Image Factory: Work Practices in MRI Units," explores the production and interpretation of examinations. This chapter documents the human relations that come together to create MRI scans. The work practices of technologists and radiologists, the two main groups responsible for producing and interpreting these images, are highlighted. Drawing on fieldwork observations and interview materials, this chapter describes the social world created in imaging units, documenting the current pressures on radiologists and technologists to accelerate their work practices and illustrating how contemporary imaging units are organized like a factory. Instead of widgets, sneakers, or articles of clothing, patients are now the objects on the assembly line. This chapter also shows how radiologists and technologists, creative actors in their own right, resist transforming their work space into an assembly line by trying to control the pace and quality of their labor through both direct and indirect means.

Chapter 5, "The Political Economy of MRI," situates the technology within a larger structural framework that takes into account the health insurance system in the Unites States and the economic structure associated with the production and marketing of MRI. In this chapter, I broaden my analytical lens to examine the links between medical visualization technologies, reimbursement practices, and profit. MRI is currently an income-generating procedure and, as such, needs to be analyzed in a way that takes this into account. This chapter traces the exchange of money in relation to MRI, following paths to and from manufacturers, radiologists, referring doctors, hospitals, health insurance companies, and patients. It also explores the connection between the production of profits and the cultural emphasis on images, arguing that current beliefs about images produced by machines make MRI and other medical imaging technologies a desirable product in U.S. markets. Patients, now positioned as consumers by health care professionals and policy makers, are active participants in the desire for and exchange of medical images. Yet caution is needed. Patients are not solely driving the acceleration and rapid diffusion of MRI technology. I discuss the tendency to define patients as consumers and how this can be used to market MRI scans in the concluding section of this chapter.

Finally, Chapter 6, "A Sacred Technology?: Theorizing Visual Knowledge in the Twenty-first Century," brings two main conclusions forward. First, this chapter discusses some social costs created by our contemporary understanding of MRI technology. The desire for scans reflects real anxieties about the quality of health care, physician skills, and increased incidence of cancer and other chronic illnesses in the United States. However, the perception that access to and use of MRI itself can produce healthier bodies encourages people to believe that this technology can also solve these larger health and social issues. Moreover, it encourages people to believe that other forms of intervention and change (e.g., political or environmental) are unnecessary. In a symbolic economy that equates the image with certainty, MRI is not just the right tool for the job. It is perceived as one of the few tools available.

Second, this chapter examines other ways of knowing about bodies once the hegemony of sight is challenged. Other clinical techniques that use touch, smell, taste, and sound to produce knowledge about the body are seriously considered, illustrating the importance of such often neglected procedures. This chapter concludes with a critical analysis of current assumptions about visibility, technology, and transparency, and offers suggestions for ways to rethink the role of MRI in health care. Although an important technique, medical imaging cannot eliminate uncertainty when offering a diagnosis, nor can it secure health in the way its supporters contend.

MRI and Medical Policies: A Cautionary Tale in the Making?

New applications and increased availability mean that we will hear more and more about MRI technology in the future. Salespeople and physicians are pushing to expand the use of MRI in health care in the United States. For example, research shows that MRI can be used to image the breast and the fetus. At this time, these areas of the body are typically imaged by ultrasound, a more cost-effective imaging modality. The approximate one-million-dollar difference in prices of the machines is seldom mentioned in the promotion of MRI technology for new applications. Such discussions also downplay issues of safety and efficiency, as well as whether scientific evidence supports the need for this increased use.

MRI is also evoked in discussions about policy and health care. In debates about universal health coverage, for example, the availability of and access to MRI machines were used to evaluate the quality of care in other nations. Individuals in the United States who opposed universal health coverage, for example, pointed to the lack of MRI machines in Canada as a way to demonstrate the superiority of the health care in the United States (Payer 1996, xiv). Journalists and politicians also used images of patients waiting in long lines for MRI exams to discourage interest in universal health care systems. This type of imagery draws on popular beliefs that equate MRI use with progress, longer life spans, and better health care. These beliefs, however, lack empirical support. Canada is ranked higher in overall health indicators such as life expectancy than the United States even though MRI technology is used less frequently there (WHO 2006). Arguments that rely on popular ideas about imaging technology will continue to be used as debates about heath insurance and universal coverage continue to reverberate. The research and analysis offered in the following chapters add a level of complexity to the dialogue concerning MRI technology.

The issues raised in *Magnetic Appeal* offer insight into broader questions about health care in the United States. The case of MRI provides a lens through which we can view how local and national cultures as well as health care organizations shape perceptions and uses of technology in medicine. The proliferation of new medical technologies and procedures will continue. It is up to us to ask difficult questions about why we feel compelled to use these medical techniques and whether they truly provide an outcome that equals not only what the technology promises but what the patient expects.

2

Painting by Numbers

The Development of Magnetic Resonance Imaging and the Visual Turn in Medicine

Magnetic resonance imaging (MRI) occupies an important symbolic space in contemporary science and popular culture. In 2003, Drs. Paul Lauterbur and Peter Mansfield were awarded the Nobel Prize in Physiology and Medicine for developing MRI technology, an event symbolizing the importance of this imaging technique to the broader scientific community. Yet while MRI is viewed as the gold standard in imaging diagnostics by policy makers and medical practitioners, it has assumed celebrity status in mass media. It is nearly impossible to read newspapers and magazines or watch television dramas such as *Law and Order* and *ER* without coming across a passage, scene, or dialogue that invokes the technology. Even the Dalai Lama (2005) singled MRI out as representative of the highest technological achievement in modern times.

Today, MRI scans and technology are central to medical practice, identities of health and illness, and social life more generally. Yet there is nothing inevitable about how MRI is presently designed or interpreted. The name of the technology, the design of the machine, and the representation of MRI data were debated and transformed during its initial development in the 1970s and immediately after its introduction into clinical medical practice in the 1980s. During these periods, research scientists, in response to culturally embedded interactions with other scientists, radiologists, and prospective patients, creatively appropriated and adapted machine design, the appearance of data output, and terminology to collectively produce what today is known as MRI.

The development of MRI technology occurred within two cultural contexts: (1) the sociotechnical turn toward visuality and (2) an emphasis on nuclear technologies and knowledge. Drawing on sociological analyses of technological innovation, this chapter addresses several critical questions. How did research scientists choose to represent the data in changing ways—from numbers to pictures of specific kinds? How did these decisions, as well as issues of professional control, relate to the broader cultural context of visualization? And, finally, how did the development of MRI relate to both scientific work in and shifting public perceptions of atomic research? This chapter shows that scientists selected from a range of possibilities to settle on and ultimately create a new technology. Their choices can only be understood through sustained discussions of larger cultural priorities and conventions.

An "Imaging" Machine?: Nuclear Physics and the Development of MRI

The ideas that provide the foundation for MRI technology are rooted in early twentieth century investigations of the internal structure of the atom and the rise of physics in scientific practice (Kevles 1987). An understanding of the centrality of nuclear physics to MRI development gives insight into how the technology produces anatomical images, and, in doing so, complicates common perceptions of it as an *imaging* apparatus. MRI, despite its current construction as a visualizing technique, does not produce anatomical images in a straightforward fashion. It has no photographic lens, nor does it use x-ray techniques to create pictures of the internal body. Instead, MRI is used to numerically measure how hydrogen nuclei absorb and release energy in response to particular frequencies.

The understanding of nuclei as a site of energy absorption and emission builds on nuclear magnetic resonance (NMR) research, a scientific area of inquiry developed in the early twentieth century. The term "nuclear magnetic resonance," coined by physicist Isidor Rabi in the 1930s, describes how nuclei of atoms absorb and release energy in response to specific frequencies when placed in a magnetic field (Wehrli 1992, 34). This process is similar to that of a tuning fork. If a person strikes a tuning fork tuned to a particular frequency, other tuning forks in the vicinity tuned to the same frequency will pick up the energy from the humming tuning fork, start to vibrate, and emit a sound. The nucleus of an atom does the same. In response to a particular frequency, the nucleus of an atom will absorb energy and then relax by emitting energy. Since different atoms (or the same atom in different environments) have different relaxation rates, this information can be used to identify the composition of a molecule; in the case of MRI, the machine measures how hydrogen nuclei absorb and release energy, which in turn provides knowledge about the placement of hydrogen atoms in the body and therefore knowledge about anatomy in the body.

The theoretical ideas that gave rise to NMR research are often traced to Austrian physicist Wolfgang Pauli's predictions about motion and magnetic fields. In 1924 Pauli theorized that the nucleus of an atom spins around on its axis. Drawing from previous research on energy, Pauli speculated that the movement of this spin must create a magnetic force around the nuclei. The portion of space around the nuclei created by this force is called a "magnetic field" or a "magnetic moment" (Grant and Harris 1996, 3).

Pauli's theoretical work sparked empirical research that documented and measured the spin of nuclei. Physicist Isidor Rabi transformed Pauli's theories into technique. In the early 1930s, Rabi designed an apparatus that used magnets and atomic beams to show that nuclear spin did actually exist (Mattson and Simon 1996, 60). After this success, Rabi continued to try and develop a way of directly measuring the magnetic moment of a nuclei. Rabi's breakthrough came after Cornelius Gorter visited his lab at Columbia University in 1937. Gorter suggested that Rabi shift the design of his machine to include an oscillator, which would create a much smaller magnetic field through the use of radio frequency waves (Mattson and Simon 1996, 66). Rabi and his team then used radio frequency waves and a changing electromagnetic field and learned that the nucleus of an atom will resonate in response to a specific frequency.[1]

Rabi's ideas and methods were crucial to the development of knowledge about NMR and still inform the construction of contemporary MRI machines. His experiments, however, focused on the detection of NMR in isolated molecules. The next two decades of research would develop the theories and tools necessary to measure NMR in bulk materials.

In the 1940s and early 1950s, physicists continued to develop their understanding of NMR, laying the foundation for later applications of NMR techniques in health care. During this time, two physicists, Edward Purcell at MIT and Felix Bloch at Stanford University, independently developed techniques that allowed for more precise measurements of NMR in bulk materials. Their work, for which they were jointly awarded the Nobel Prize

---

[1] There are two ways to measure nuclear magnetic resonance. The first is to vary the external magnetic field while holding the frequency of the oscillator constant. The second is to hold the external magnetic field constant while varying the frequency of the oscillator. In Rabi's first resonance experiment he used the first method. After this, however, he switched to the second method (Mattson and Simon 1996, 66 and 117).

in Physics in 1952, provided a more in-depth understanding of the way the spin of nuclei absorbed and released energy (Office of Technology Assessment [OTA] 1984, 4). Bloch, in addition to this work, also developed a series of equations that produced two different measurements, T1 and T2 relaxation times; these relaxation times provided nuanced information about the absorption and emission of energy by protons (Mattson and Simon 1996, 353). Other physicists, such as Nicolaas Bloembergen and Erwin Hahn, created further techniques and theories that helped turn this relatively theoretical knowledge into applied knowledge; their innovations enabled the production of tools useful beyond the physics laboratory.

While efforts to use this technology for medical diagnosis did not occur until the early 1970s, several crucial shifts helped move the technology from research science to clinical practice (Kevles 1997, 177; Lauterbur 1996, 447). Nuclear magnetic resonance, now a commercially available technology, expanded into the realm of chemistry in the late 1950s (Blume 1992, 191). This move started the slow transformation of NMR into a visualizing technology—one that produced pictorial representations as well as numerical values. Chemists primarily used NMR to identify the structure of molecules. Research showed that each type of molecule had its own unique frequency at which resonance occurs. The property of resonance at a particular frequency allowed chemists to use NMR as a way to identify the types of molecules present in a particular substance thereby analyzing the exact makeup of complex substances.

Chemists represented the information produced by NMR as lines with peaks on a graph. This form of representation was used to represent different frequencies at which resonance occurred and became the standard way of portraying the information within chemistry.

Beyond chemistry, some researchers began using NMR techniques to measure blood flow and muscle movement in live animals. This work, however, remained marginal. It was in the 1970s that NMR research firmly shifted to the realm of medical applications.

Constructing a Medical Technology

During the early 1970s, American physician Raymond Damadian, American chemist Paul Lauterbur, and British physicist Peter Mansfield each independently tinkered with existing NMR techniques, looking for ways to extend its applications. Demonstrating how science is a cultural practice, each man's research was shaped by his professional training and his location within broader cultural contexts.

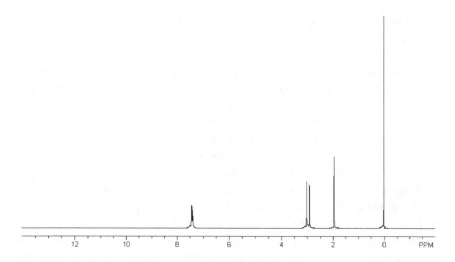

A high-resolution NMR spectrum. *Source*: J. C. Poutsma, College of William and Mary.

Damadian, a physician at the Downstate Medical Center in New York, pioneered the use of NMR in medical practice. Damadian experimented with using NMR techniques to diagnose cancer. He hoped that the new procedure could replace surgery and biopsies in cancer care.

Damadian's choice of cancer was not arbitrary. It was shaped by the culture of the early 1970s in the United States when cancer was constructed as a central social problem. In 1970 the U.S. Senate evaluated the state of cancer research and recommended that the diagnosis and treatment of cancer should become a national priority. In his State of the Union message on January 22, 1971, President Richard Nixon proclaimed that "The time has come in America when the same kind of concentrated effort that split the atom and took man to the moon should be turned toward curing this dread disease. Let us make a total national commitment to achieve this goal." At the end of that year, Nixon signed the National Cancer Act and encouraged researchers to come up with a cure for cancer in five years. The visibility of this legislative act was high; the popular press featured articles on what became known as Nixon's "War on Cancer." Research money became available and scientists were enrolled to find ways to detect and understand cancer.

As an American physician, Damadian's clinical attention, like many U.S. scientists and physicians at this time, was focused primarily on cancer. In an effort to develop a diagnostic procedure for cancer that did not require surgery, Damadian used NMR to analyze differences between cancerous and normal tissues. Building on previous research that showed cancer cells

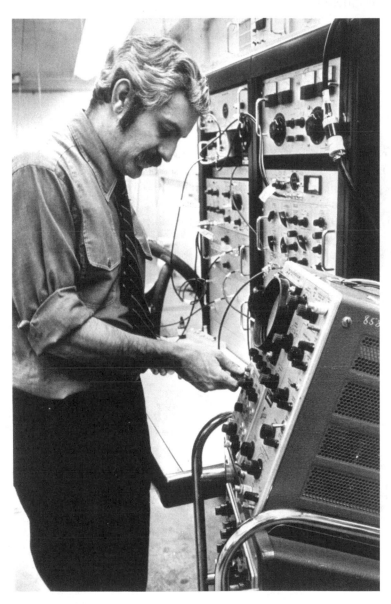

Damadian at NMR scope. *Source*: FONAR Corporation.

filled with water, Damadian hypothesized that "it would be possible to detect the difference between a cancerous cell and a normal cell purely from
its chemistry" and decided to use NMR techniques to do so (Kleinfield
1985, 18). In his research, Damadian placed normal and cancerous tissue
from rats in a NMR apparatus. The technology measured the time it took
for the hydrogen nuclei in the tissue to absorb and release the energy from
the radio waves. Damadian found that cancerous and normal tissues had
different measurements (i.e., T1 and T2 relaxation times). Hopeful that he
had discovered an important diagnostic technique, Damadian published
this research in the March 19, 1971 issue of *Science* under the title "Tumor
Detection by Nuclear Magnetic Resonance" (Damadian 1971).

Damadian also filed a patent that described a full-body NMR scanner.
The patent application "Apparatus and Method for Detecting Cancer in Tissue" was filed on March 17, 1972, and eventually issued in 1974 (Mattson
and Simon 1996, 668). The patent covered the use of NMR on both excised

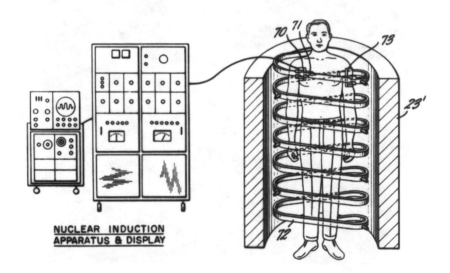

3,789,832

SHEET 2 OF 2

NUCLEAR INDUCTION
APPARATUS & DISPLAY

FIG. 2

Damadian's patent filed on March 17, 1972. *Source*: FONAR Corporation.

tissue samples and living human bodies (Mattson and Simon 1996, A14–A19). In both the article and the patent, Damadian makes no mention of turning the NMR data into an anatomical picture; the information obtained about the body through NMR technology was outputted as numbers.

Damadian's article in *Science* sparked great interest at a time when concern about cancer was prevalent among the public, government officials, and scientific communities. Researchers grabbed hold of Damadian's work and tried to replicate his results. In early September 1971, Leon Saryan worked on this project at NMR Specialties in New Kensington, Pennsylvania (Hollis 1987, 138). While at this laboratory, chemist Paul Lauterbur watched Saryan's research and imagined different uses for the information produced by NMR (Lauterbur 1996, 447). Describing his impression of Saryan's work, Lauterbur (1986, 1899) explained:

Although there were clear differences between samples taken from rat hepatomas and those removed from other tissues of the animal, there seemed to be no plausible explanation for the differences, nor did it seem likely to me that one more method of characterizing biopsy specimens would have much medical impact. However, even normal tissues differed markedly among themselves in NMR relaxation times, and I wondered whether there might be some way to noninvasively map out such quantities within the body.

Intrigued, Lauterbur continued to think about how normal tissue relaxation times differed. He decided this information could be used to make a new technology—one that would create anatomical pictures, or what Lauterbur referred to as "maps" of the inner body. In what is now recognized as an important innovation, Lauterbur decided to use a *gradient*, which is a coil that creates a second magnetic field, in addition to a large magnet, to produce this type of information. This technique initially created numerical data that demonstrated the location of the signal emitted by nuclei. This data, Lauterbur suggested, could then be coded and transformed into an anatomical picture of the internal body.

The decision to produce anatomical images shifted NMR use in an important new direction even as it simultaneously drew on what Charles Goodwin (1994) would call Lauterbur's professional vision. In his analysis of archeologists and expert witnesses, Goodwin shows how professionals learn, through a process of interaction with colleagues, the material world, and events, to order and represent the world in an occupationally specific manner. This "professional vision" shapes how one highlights, ignores, and thus portrays aspects of objects and relations. Lauterbur, as a chemist, learned through interactions with colleagues to organize and produce the physical world using a particular set of methods and representational strategies. Although chemists produce and interpret other modes of representation, visual displays, such as three-dimensional models and graphs, are embedded in their discipline and are commonly used. Chemists, for example, portrayed the information produced through NMR techniques in visual form, representing the frequencies as lines on a graph. They did not primarily work with the data as numbers. Lauterbur's professional vision emphasized the use of visual depictions, and, in doing so, facilitated his ability to translate the data into graphic form.

Lauterbur discussed the proposed visual output through the use of cartographical metaphors. Trained as a chemist, Lauterbur described the image as a mathematical representation of spatial information. Lauterbur used words like *map* to describe the output, and when he used terms like *picture* and *image*, he defined them in mathematical terms (Lauterbur 1973; Lauterbur et al. 1975). For example, Lauterbur writes, "an image of an object may be defined as a graphical representation of the spatial distribution of one or more of its properties" (Lauterbur 1973, 190). Here, the image is primarily described as a "graphical representation" that visually shows the spatial distribution of hydrogen nuclei, and its meaning is not assumed to be evident.

Lauterbur's choice of cartographical metaphors stands in sharp contrast to the way physicians and patients now describe the image. Today, language that highlights the relation of the image to pictures of the anatomical body are often used in clinical practice, while language that calls attention to maps and spatiality is less common (see, e.g., Beaulieu 2002; Joyce 2005). This linguistic difference occurs in part because of the broader recognition of the centrality of images to contemporary life as visualizing technologies such as cameras, computers, video games, and picture-producing cell phones become more common. Medical imaging technologies such as ultrasound and computed tomography (CT) technology—which were in initial stages of diffusion in the early 1970s—are routinely used in clinical practice and are a crucial part of this trend.

However, the linguistic difference between Lauterbur and practicing physicians is not simply a matter of time (i.e., then versus now). This difference also shows how professional contexts shape which metaphors are used to describe representations of the body. Anne Beaulieu (2002) demonstrates this point in her work on brain scans. Beaulieu's research shows that neuroscientists in research laboratories use narratives that emphasize the mathematical components of brain images. In contrast, pictorial metaphors are typically used in clinical practice to describe the same sort of scan (Beaulieu 2002, 63). Thus, there are multiple ways to discuss anatomical images, and professional and cultural contexts support the choice of particular rhetorical practices over others.

Lauterbur wrote his ideas about NMR and gradients in his notebook on September 2, 1971, and had this entry witnessed (Mattson and Simon 1996, 714). Securing additional recognition of his contribution, Lauterbur then published a paper in the March 16, 1973 issue of *Nature*. In this piece, Lauterbur argued for the use of anatomical representations as the form of display for the information obtained by the technology. He also proposed the name "zeugmatography" for his invention and called the images produced "zeugmatograms." Zeugmatography, derived from the Greek word *zeugma*, means "that which is used for joining." Emphasizing the technique rather than the output, the term symbolizes how the magnet and the gradients "join together" to create information about the inner body (Lauterbur 1973, 190).

With this publication, Lauterbur entered the public scientific dialogue about possible new uses for NMR techniques. Lauterbur was not the only scientist, however, to imagine extending the technology to create spatial information. In the United Kingdom, physicist Peter Mansfield also envisioned using NMR in this manner, but with a different target. In contrast to Lauterbur, Mansfield wanted to use the technology to map inert matter, not human anatomy. As a trained physicist, Mansfield studied not human anatomy but rigid matter such as crystals. Mansfield hoped that NMR techniques could be extended to produce spatial information about this type of substance.

Mansfield and his colleague Peter Grannell published their ideas about using NMR techniques to produce spatial data in a letter called "NMR Diffraction in Solids?" in *The Journal of Physics C*, an academic journal dedicated to reporting new solid state physics theory and research, in 1973. In this letter Mansfield and Grannell explained how gradients could be used to obtain spatial information about solids such as crystals. They made no mention of using this technique on human or animal tissue, nor did they discuss turning the information into a picture.

Mansfield did speculate about using visual representations, however, when he presented his ideas in September 1973 at the first Specialized Colloque AMPERE in Poland.[2] Ulrich Haeberlen, a participant at the

---

[2] The AMPERE group was founded in 1952 in France with the aim of promoting dialogue between European research laboratories and aiding scientists in difficult economic or political conditions. Since the 1950s, the group has sponsored numerous specialized colloques, summer schools and institutes, forums, and workshops dedicated to research on magnetic resonances, optics, magnetic resonance imaging, as well as the development of related methodologies and technologies. The AMPERE group's website is http://www.ampere.ethz.ch/.

conference, remembers, "And Peter Mansfield, what did he talk about? He began with reflection symmetry in sequences but soon turned to NMR diffractometry. In retrospect, he talked and speculated about spin imaging and actually showed pictures of phantoms!" (Grant and Harris 1996, 118). Haeberlen's excitement here refers to Mansfield's reflection about the potential use of images to represent NMR data. Although unknown at this time, the turn toward the visual would prove to be a key component of the medical device eventually developed for use in clinical practice and embraced by popular culture.

Mansfield's presentation prompted his introduction to Lauterbur's research. After Mansfield delivered his lecture, a member of the audience "stood up during the question period and asked Mansfield if he knew of Paul Lauterbur's recent paper which presented the idea of using NMR to form images" (Grant and Harris 1996, 387). Mansfield hadn't heard of Lauterbur, and when he returned home he looked up his work. He noted the similarities between their ideas and experimented with transforming Lauterbur's idea of using NMR to visualize anatomy into a viable technology.

In this early stage of research and development, Damadian, Lauterbur, and Mansfield all worked on extending NMR technology use. While each man's professional location shaped his initial work with NMR—Damadian, an American doctor, focused on cancer; Mansfield, a physicist, concentrated on crystals; and Lauterbur, a chemist, imagined using NMR techniques to produce pictorial representations—their research agendas expanded and changed in response to exchanges with each other. All three scientists incorporated Lauterbur and Damadian's insistence on using NMR technology to produce knowledge about the human body and Lauterbur and Mansfield's desire to create spatial information into their research. Each changed their investigations to focus on these issues.

Standardizing Terminology, Representational Practices, and Machine Design

Throughout the mid- to late 1970s the desire to create a medical technology out of existing NMR techniques gained momentum, and the circle of researchers involved expanded. Research teams in Japan, the United Kingdom, and the United States worked on transforming Damadian, Lauterbur, and Mansfield's insights into a viable medical technology. As research moved into more laboratories and sites, scientists negotiated the name, design, and mode of representation of the technique. In this early stage of innovation, decisions about data output and machine design were primarily shaped by competing professional visions of the research scientists intimately involved in MRI development. While access to funding and institutional structures enabled their work, the research scientists' expectations and training significantly impacted their research developments.[3]

During this round of innovation and development, the new, extended community of researchers quietly rejected Lauterbur's proposed name for the emergent technology. While some scientists initially adopted *zeugmatography* to talk about the new technology, most continued to use NMR—an already familiar term that highlighted connections to its scientific roots in nuclear physics and chemistry (Hoult 1979; Kumar, Welti, and Ernst 1975; Lauterbur et al. 1975).

Scientists also rejected the idea that the numerical data was not of interest in itself. In his early work, Lauterbur argued that the picture was *the* component of NMR data to be produced and used. Despite his insistence, scientists continued to publish the data as both an array of numbers and an anatomical image (Lauterbur 1986; Mallard et al. 1979; Mansfield and Maudsley 1977). Some researchers thought that the number values provided a degree of specificity that was lost when these values were turned into parts of an image. Damadian, explaining this belief to me in an interview, noted, "We thought that an actual knowledge of the T1 and T2 [measurements], rather than translating it into a pixel brightness, would give an additional quantitative handle on how big the differences were" (Damadian 2000). The numerical measurements might provide additional knowledge about a person's health that would be unavailable once these values were translated into components of an image.

In addition to deciding to *produce* images, researchers also had to figure out the *appearance* of image content. NMR research scientists typically had little experience working with anatomical images in medicine. Still operating in the laboratory, they did not have to answer to the needs and expectations of professions that routinely worked with images or patients. These men, free to tinker with the representational form, chose vibrant, rainbow colors, such as green, yellow, and red, to represent the inner body (Damadian et al. 1978; Edelstein et al. 1981; Mallard et al. 1979). Resembling Andy Warhol or Roy Lichtenstein's bright color prints, the scientists' choices mirrored the aesthetics of popular art and television in the 1970s, a decade known for psychedelic colors and artifacts such as mood rings, lava lamps, and Pop Rocks candy (Panati 1991).

These decisions about data portrayal subsequently shaped decisions about machine design. Representational practices were built into the

---

[3] For further discussion of the financial relations that structured MRI development, see Blume (1992, 192–217).

design of the machine, and early scanners were made so that both forms of representation—numerical and visual—could be easily accessed. Engineer Larry Crooks noted in correspondence with me that the University of California at San Francisco (UCSF) scanner "had a track ball [a belly-up mouse] that let one position a cursor on the image and read the intensity number from any location. There were also functions that would calculate the average and standard deviation of the numbers from any closed region one could draw on the image" (Crooks 2000). Additionally, the scanners developed by other research teams were designed to allow users to move easily between the numerical and anatomical forms of representation.

By the end of the 1970s, the research teams had arrived at a working consensus about the name of the technology, the representation of the data, and the machine design. The common name for the technology was *nuclear magnetic resonance imaging,* or *NMR.* The display of the data included printouts of multicolor images and arrays of numbers, and machines were designed to produce this output. The chemists, physicists, and research physicians who worked on the technique drew on professional knowledge and exchanges with each other to stabilize the features of NMR imaging. In doing so, the scientists created a new cultural product—a medical technology called *NMR imaging*—and an understanding of the inner body as T1 and T2 relaxation times, represented in both numerical and multicolored, visual form. The name NMR imaging highlighted the connections between the new technology and its scientific roots in nuclear physics and chemistry while the production of both visual and numerical data created a new way of "knowing" the internal body. As potential users expanded to include practicing physicians and potential patients, these choices would be actively challenged.

MRI Machines in Clinical Practice

NMR imaging technology entered clinical practice in the 1980s. When first introduced, it was unclear which medical specialty should control NMR imaging technology. It could have, for example, been placed in nuclear medicine or pathology departments. Nuclear medicine physicians or pathologists are trained to understand the body through a detailed knowledge of chemistry and nuclear physics and are able to interpret the biochemical, numerical information produced by NMR techniques. NMR, however, also produces anatomical pictures. As such, a link to radiology could be argued. Radiologists order and produce the body through anatomical pictures and are today considered experts in image interpretation. The diverse features of NMR imaging technology—it produced both numerical and visual information—meant that the machine could potentially be placed in different departments.

During the early 1980s research scientists and nuclear medicine physicians publicly discussed machine placement, and some expressed concern about radiologists' bias toward images. John Mallard, for example, questioned radiologists' ability to interpret numerical information, noting that:

> The human body is extremely complex. When . . . we first attempt to image a new property such as proton magnetic resonance, there is bound to be difficulty in interpreting the results . . . With this in mind, we have carried out a biological back-up program of T1 measurement on normal and pathological tissues to ease the problem of image interpretation and to find pointers toward the most fruitful fields for the application of NMR imaging. (Mallard, quoted in Blume 1992, 218)

Nuclear medicine physicians also challenged radiologists' emphasis on images. Paul Lauterbur (2000), in my interview with him, recalls:

> People in nuclear medicine, I had heard say about that time, said that radiologists could not be trusted with nuclear magnetic resonance imaging. It was too complicated for them. People in nuclear medicine were used to thinking about chemistry and complex physics while radiologists just looked at fuzzy pictures.

Thus, there was concern that radiologists would ignore "the most fruitful fields" of NMR, the biochemical information, and focus only on the visual component.

These expressions of unease remained minor though. NMR imaging, despite the potential connections to nuclear medicine and pathology and the misgivings of some scientists, eventually became part of radiology units in many countries.

Changes within radiology and medicine provided institutional support for this decision. Professional radiology organizations, such as the Radiological Society of North America (RSNA) and the American College of Radiology (ACR), reached peak membership numbers in the 1970s (Linton 1997; RSNA 2005a). Drawing on their expanding membership base, these organizations actively lobbied to gain control over imaging interpretation. As the ACR Board Chairman Robert Wise noted, "It has taken us a decade to build our specialty up to the point where we can contemplate providing the radiologic services needed by the American people. This puts us in a position to assert that radiology should be done by radiologists where we are available to do it" (Wise, quoted in Linton 1997, 86). Legally, any licensed medical doctor has the right to interpret medical images, and radiologists lost revenue and status when other physicians did visual interpretation work. Instead of directly challenging laws that allowed any licensed medical doctor to interpret medical images, radiology organizations questioned the ability of other physicians to "read" images correctly. This move was successful in many countries and contributed to the idea that radiologists are *the* professional authorities over image interpretation.

In the United States, radiologists gained even more independence and control. In the early 1970s the ACR encouraged radiologists to "gain independent practice status in their hospitals" (Linton 1997, 80). This move allowed radiologists to operate in hospitals but maintain control over their fees and income. Initially resisting, the American Hospital Association acquiesced to this demand and, due in part to lobbying efforts by the ACR, stopped pursuing legislature to "recapture" radiology.

The 1970s, a key decade in the rise of radiology, also witnessed an increase in the range and number of imaging technologies available. In this decade, techniques such as CT and ultrasound became part of clinical practice and increased physicians' choice of imaging techniques. X-ray had previously been the only imaging apparatus commonly used. The increased range and presence of anatomical pictures in medicine, coupled with the expansion of radiologists' authority and prestige, supported the plausibility of placing NMR imaging technology in radiology units. The high cost and large size of NMR machines further ensured that private physicians would not purchase their own machines, cementing the technology's initial placement in hospital-based radiology departments.

Radiologists Shape Machine Output and Design

The placement of NMR imaging in radiology departments was a crucial decision that opened dialogue between the existing technique and radiologists' professional vision. As noted earlier, *professional vision* refers to the way individuals are trained through interaction processes to code and highlight the world in an occupationally specific manner (Goodwin 1994). Radiologists are disciplined, through interaction with other physicians, medical textbooks, and imaging machines, to represent and interpret their area of focus—the body, health, and illness—as black and white images. They do not work with the body in numerical form.

The dialogue between radiologists' professional vision and NMR imaging consequently resulted in two major changes in the appearance of the data. First, the practice of printing out both the array of numbers and anatomical pictures ceased soon after NMR imaging was placed in radiology units. Instead of representing NMR data as both numbers and images, the data was now presented solely in image form.

Developers of MRI recall how radiologists' emphasis on pictures shaped decisions about representation practices. During an interview, Mallard remembered, "Our very first mouse image, we did actually publish it with all of the numbers and then we showed a color version of it, converting those numbers into the different bands of color that we decided to use. You could see an abnormality in the mouse from the color change. You could see it in the numbers as well, but radiologists don't think that way . . . Radiologists just weren't interested in the numbers. They never have been" (Mallard 2000). For Mallard, both forms of display—the array of numbers and the anatomical picture of the body—reveal the location of abnormalities, and it was radiologists' preferences that shaped the turn toward the image.

Larry Crooks, a member of the UCSF NMR imaging research laboratory, also discussed the importance of radiologists' professional vision in decisions about data appearance. Crooks explained that the image came to dominate because, "We were in the radiology department. The docs make their living looking at images" (Crooks 2000).

The same pattern occurred when CT imaging was introduced to radiology units in the early 1970s. Similar to NMR technology, CT scanners do not "take a picture" of the internal body; instead, they numerically measure the amount of x-ray absorbed by tissues. Mathematical formulas then transform numbers into visual representations of the internal body. Early scanners printed out both the array of numbers and the anatomical picture for each exam (Kevles 1997, 161), and initial articles that reported CT scans included both the numerical and pictorial representations of the information (Ambrose 1973).

As with NMR imaging, the practice of printing both numerical and visual forms of representations ended shortly after CT technology was placed under the jurisdiction of radiologists and radiology units. Calling attention to the "radiology" effect, historian Bettyann Kevles (1997, 161) notes that "Few, if any, radiologists ever looked at the numbers," and the practice of printing out numerical data ceased after the incorporation of CT scanners into radiology units.

In the case of NMR imaging technology, the professional vision of radiologists caused a second change in data appearance by transforming the content of the image from multicolor to gray scale. The machine design was altered so that the final product was not a multicolor picture. Numerical values were coded into shades of gray, and the resulting images were printed on black and white film. NMR machines now produced the body as a black and white image, and representations of the body as arrays of reds, yellows, and blues disappeared from clinical practice.[4]

Mallard (2000) recalls, "Our first images were in color. The interesting thing is that all the radiologists couldn't abide by colors. They were used to gray scale on their x-rays and they wanted gray scale. So we put gray scale. Everybody else went to gray scale and color was dropped." Paul Lauterbur (2000) also remembers the importance of the professional expectations of radiologists in the process of standardizing the color of the image. He explained, "The general practice of using gray scale came about because radiologists were used to such images from x-rays and CAT scanning."

Radiologists prefer gray-scale images in part because they are trained to interpret this type of picture. To switch to a new mode of image appearance, such as multicolor or an image printed in a different tint, would require a significant retraining of the eye and the mind. This time investment is impractical in the busy world of everyday medical practice, and physicians resist such changes. In addition, since radiologists already worked with CT and x-ray images, supporting technologies such as printers and film accommodated the use of gray scale. As Lauterbur (2000) points out, "their systems for recording and reproducing images used black and white film" and to change to other colors would be costly.

Radiologists also prefer images in hues of one color because this form of representation allows them to identify subtle anatomical changes. As physician Damadian (2000) explains, "When you start using [different] colors, you can go from one region of pixel brightness to another region where the difference between the two regions numerically is small, but you code one a yellow and the other a blue. There's this huge discontinuity on the picture, which on the gray scale would be a negligible transition." This abrupt change in color can suggest the difference between the two areas is very large, when in fact it is small. It can, as engineer Crooks

---

[4] The early use of color images continues to haunt some contemporary MRI scans. Occasionally, a very low signal is produced during an MRI exam. Some scanners, using a coding practice left over from earlier machine designs, still translate this signal into the color red. The low signal thus appears as red dribbles above and below the anatomy in the image. Scientists jokingly call these distortions "bleeding artifacts," using humor to trouble cultural boundaries that distinguish between the image as inanimate and the body as life (Crooks 2000).

(2000) suggests, "trick the eye into believing two close numbers are very different, because they are different colors in the image." This "tricking" of an eye may cause physicians to misinterpret the exam because subtle transitions between parts of the body are not highlighted. The color chosen, of course, could be any shade; it does not have to be shades of gray. The use of printers and film to produce black and white CT and x-ray images, coupled with radiologists' already disciplined vision, reinforced the decision to choose this color over other possibilities.

Finally, as expectations of users are "built in" to technologies, the radiologists' interpretive practices also shaped subsequent changes in machine design (Bijker 1995). New machines were crafted in ways that made it more difficult for physicians to move between the numerical values and the image. Now machines immediately produced and displayed anatomical pictures on the computer screen. While the quantitative information was often still available, it was no longer visible on the screen or printed as part of the exam process. It required a series of software commands to become apparent. Gradually, numerical data disappeared from clinical practice.

Anti-Nuclear Movements and Changes in Terminology

If the expectations of radiologists significantly altered both data representation and the machine itself, American perceptions of the term *nuclear* also presented a crucial transformative force. The name of the new technology—NMR imaging—was challenged once introduced into clinical medical practice in the early 1980s. A heightened consciousness about the problems associated with both nuclear power plants and nuclear weapons marked this time period. The anti–nuclear power plant movement in the United States had been building momentum since the 1970s. On March 28, 1979, the Three Mile Island Nuclear Plant released radioactive material into the air. Although not the first such "accident," it was the first to receive significant attention, and it helped mobilize the "No Nukes" campaign. Many proposals for new plants were strongly contested. Between 1977 and 1989, for example, over 3,500 people were arrested in protests against the nuclear power plant in Seabrook, New Hampshire, alone (Zinn 1995, 600–601).

In addition to the anti–nuclear power plant movement, other groups, such as the Nuclear Weapons Freeze Campaign, actively challenged the proliferation of nuclear arms in the United States and the Union of Soviet Socialist Republics (U.S.S.R.). The actions of groups like the Nuclear Weapons Freeze Campaign, the Committee for a Sane Nuclear Policy

(SANE), and others successfully challenged the legitimacy of nuclear weapons in the United States. In 1982, nuclear freeze resolutions were on many city and state ballots, and there was a widespread awareness of the dangerousness of the nuclear arms race (Gusterson 1996, 169).

It was during the height of this nuclear national consciousness that NMR imaging made its way into American hospitals. The symbolic connection between the name of the new technology and nuclear weapons and power plants reverberated throughout clinical practice. What emerged was a cultural impossibility of separating the word *nuclear* in "nuclear magnetic resonance imaging" from the danger associated with the global nuclear social context. As Mallard (2000) recalls, "Nuclear was associated with bombs and wars and God knows what." Concerned about this negative association, U.S. physician Dr. Alexander Margulis promoted a new name, *magnetic resonance imaging* or *MRI*, and the American College of Radiology supported it (Axel 2006). The new name was quickly adopted worldwide.[5]

Emerging from local political contexts within the United States, the transformation in terminology also signals shifts in the larger cultural milieu. The linguistic change from NMR to MRI technology, while a direct response to negative public perceptions of nuclear technologies, occurred as physics lost cultural and institutional prestige. As Donna Haraway (1997) and others have shown, the influence and prestige of physics and nuclear research waned in the 1980s as biology, genetics, and imaging techniques gained prominence in both scientific and popular cultures.[6] Moreover, the removal of the word *nuclear* not only distanced the technology from its roots in physics but also made it more difficult to imagine MRI as a producer of information about one's nuclei. In contrast, the new name, magnetic resonance imaging, through its emphasis on images, discursively transformed the machine into an *imaging* technique. In doing so, it aligned the new technology with the visual and signaled the increasing importance of visualization and biomedicine in the late twentieth century.

---

[5] Some scientists and physicians outside of the United States still resist this change. In my research, European physicians and scientists spontaneously discussed how the name of NMR imaging became MRI imaging, using terms such as "self-indulgence" and "American silliness" to describe the change. These scientists expressed impatience with the way the rest of the world is expected to adjust to what is happening in the United States. Their critique calls attention to the technoscientific forms of imperialism that structure the production of new technologies.

[6] See, e.g., Park Doing's analysis (2003) of labor practices in a synchrotron laboratory. Doing shows how biologists slowly replaced physicists in scheduling and priority hierarchies, and, in doing so, radically restructured knowledge production in the laboratory.

From Nuclear to Visual: Shifting Cultural Imaginations

The development of MRI technology illustrates the importance of culture to scientific innovation. The decisions about machine design, output, and name were profoundly shaped by changes in public understandings of nuclear technologies and knowledge and by what I call the "visual turn."

Throughout the twentieth century, the ability to technologically transform daily life into visual form significantly expanded (Clarke 2004; Mirzoeff 1998; Sturken and Cartwright 2001). Older technologies such as film, photography, and television were joined by new technologies such as video cassette recorders (VCRs), cable television, computers, and video games in the 1970s and 1980s. In addition, a "visual arms race" occurred as older, public space visual technologies such as film tried to regain declining audiences through publicity about and use of techniques such as widescreen movies and high quality stereophonic sound. The expansion in the range of and accessibility to visual technologies as home cameras and computers became more affordable helped render the translation of life into image form common practice.

Technological innovation in science and medicine was part of this broader tendency to translate the world into technovisual terms. Throughout the 1950s, 1960s, and 1970s, many researchers independently worked to create new technologies that would produce the body as anatomical pictures. This labor resulted in the now familiar imaging techniques such as ultrasound, computed tomography (CT), single photon emission computed tomography (SPECT), and MRI (Blume 1992; Kevles 1997; Wobarst 1999). The U.S. government recognized the importance of images to contemporary medicine: On December 29, 2000, the National Institutes of Health (NIH) created the National Institute of Biomedical Imaging and Bioengineering—the only institute of health dedicated solely to technology. The majority of institutes are organized around a particular disease or area in the body.

MRI and other medical imaging researchers' work thus tapped into and helped produce the centrality of images in modern life. The tendency toward visualization provided the technological support and cultural recognition needed to produce medical imaging as a desirable practice. The invention of new medical imaging technologies, in turn, aided visualization by producing more visual artifacts for consumption in scientific practice and popular culture.

The content of visual displays, of course, varies. Medical practice and popular culture have their own representational practices that at times overlap and at other times diverge. In the 1970s, MRI scans, for example, converged with popular culture aesthetics. Television shows like *The Partridge Family*, the continued presence of pop art, and fashions associated with musical genres such as glam rock and disco transformed the world into vibrant and at times psychedelic hues. The research scientists working on MRI development also chose bright, flashy colors to represent the inner body—a decision that resonated with the aesthetics of popular culture.

In the early 1980s, however, MRI representaional practices deviated from popular culture practices. As the 1970s waned, popular culture changed to accommodate new stylistic forms. In the 1980s, colors became more muted, denim made a comeback, and shows such as *Geraldo, Oprah, Cheers*, and *Miami Vice* took over the television screen. While the final choice of gray-scale images shared some of the oversimplified realism that infused much of the decade's popular culture, the final decisions about MRI output diverged from other stylistic practices like the use of color and a tendency toward excess. Instead, the final form of MRI scans emerged from radiologists' professional training and existing medical representational practices.

As gray-scale images, MRI examinations were made to fit an already established medical visual culture. Thus, the visual turn responds to local and specific aesthetic forms. The trend toward visualization has occurred across many milieus, but it is not monolithic. There have emerged multiple visual cultures—each with its own normative practices.

Conclusion

The science of MRI technology is based on theories of nuclear physics, specifically those concerning atomic resonance and magnetic spin. As a tool for chemists and physicists, the technology's output was numerical data that could then be interpreted as information on the chemical makeup of inert matter. Encountering an open terrain of possibilities, Raymond Damadian, Paul Lauterbur, and Peter Mansfield, along with others, worked in different ways to extend existing NMR techniques into new areas.

In the next round of research and development, researchers in Japan, the United Kingdom, and the United States crafted machines to produce both numerical data and multicolor images. These scientists, trained in a range of disciplines such as physics, chemistry, and engineering, explored the potential of both numerical and visual information. Unhampered by ties to clinical medicine, these researchers chose colors such as red, yellow, and blue to depict image content. The multicolor image aligned with the aesthetic practices of popular culture during the 1970s and mirrored the tendency to represent the world in bright, psychedelic colors.

Two significant changes occurred when the technology was introduced to clinical practice in the 1980s. First, the word *nuclear* was dropped from its name. This change occurred against a backdrop of negative public perceptions of nuclear power, nuclear weapons, and exposure to radiation. The name change not only distanced the technology from its nuclear roots but also aligned the technology more firmly with images and visuality.

Second, what the machine produced was altered. What started as a dual output of easily accessible numerical data and brightly colored images created from that data was changed to a standardized production of gray-scale images. This change occurred because radiologists became the most common users of the technology. Radiologists did not work with the body in numerical form nor did they interpret multicolor images. Instead, they translated and understood the body as gray-scale pictures. Responding to the professional expectations of radiologists and the standardized appearance of images produced by established technologies such as x-ray, CT, and ultrasound, MRI machines were designed to manufacture the body exclusively in shades of gray. While this choice shared the tendency of 1980s popular culture to produce the world through the lens of simplistic realism, it diverged from other popular culture practices that emphasized color and excess. The difference between images created for popular culture and MRI examinations shows that there are multiple visual aesthetic practices and that the visual turn is anything but monolithic.

Professional training and vision significantly shaped choices about the appearance of MRI data. However, the decision to represent data output solely as an anatomical picture is also related to the broader context of visualization and the visual turn. Computer hardware and software innovations provided the technoscientific support required to produce anatomical images that ultimately contribute to the trend toward visualization. Without these supporting technologies, the use of images as the representational form would be next to impossible. The proliferation of images in all areas of daily life further supplied the cultural familiarity needed to position MRI examinations as recognizable and desirable.

Paying attention to visualization also shows the cultural role of images in professional development and power. Radiologists gained authority and wealth throughout the 1970s and 1980s as imaging technologies were developed and perceived as needed. In the United States, radiologists now earn as much, if not more, than other lucrative medical specialties such as cardiac surgeons (RSNA 2003). Granted, factors such as lobbying efforts by professional organizations such as the Radiological Society of North

America (RSNA) and insurance reimbursement policies contribute to the prestige of radiologists. However, the cultural emphasis on images helped legitimize the work of radiologists and secure the status of their profession.

Science and technology studies scholar Nelly Oudshoorn (2003, 12) recommends more analysis of "the broader cultural dimensions of human agency" in studies of technological change. Such dimensions include representational conventions, belief systems, and the formation of identities. Following Oudshoorn's lead, this chapter demonstrates how the development of MRI relates to contemporary visual aesthetic practices and how radiologists, a newly formed professional identity, benefit from and contribute to the visual turn. Scientists creatively select, adapt, and appropriate information and ideas from a range of possibilities to produce new technologies. The decisions they make in the course of producing these technologies, especially in the case of the medical imaging, are intimately connected to the larger cultural context of visualization.

3

Seeing Is Believing

The Transformation of MRI Examinations into Authoritative Knowledge

"Bodies: The Exhibition," a traveling museum exhibit, displays room after room of body parts in display cases and preserved full bodies in poses set throughout the exhibition halls. When one enters the exhibit, written on the wall are the words, "The study of human anatomy has always operated on a basic principle—to see is to know." The "educational" premise is that visitors will learn about health and disease by seeing the muscles, nervous system, organs, and bones of dissected bodies. In the final exhibition room, displays of physical bodies give way to displays on medical treatments for illnesses, which includes a lengthy discussion of MRI technology. It is one of few technologies mentioned specifically by name in the exhibit; most medical branches and interventions are mentioned in broad categories (e.g., genomics or pharmaceuticals). As a result, the exhibit positions MRI as an advanced diagnostic technology—one that allows people to "see" and thus "know" the body. Within the exhibit narrative, this knowledge is perceived as crucial to healing.

The presentation of MRI in this exhibit is indicative of the highly privileged position that the technology occupies in relation to other technologies and to the goals of medicine: the identification and cure of disease. Similar claims for MRI are often made in sources as diverse as popular science books, television dramas, news articles, museum displays, and Hollywood films. Such claims rely in part on cultural beliefs that link seeing with knowing.

Far removed from its historical roots in atomic research, MRI technology is now a visualization technology—one understood to transform the inner body into an anatomical picture. As such, it produces a cultural artifact important to contemporary questions of identity, truth, and health.

This chapter demonstrates how popular accounts produce and magnify particular ideas about MRI examinations while marginalizing alternative ways of understanding them. This chapter identifies three common rhetorical practices used to discuss MRI in the news media, science exhibits, and popular science books: (1) MRI reveals the body and produces health; (2) MRI is compared to other medical techniques and is declared to be superior; and (3) MRI is portrayed as an agent and is represented as a machine that speaks and acts. Such narratives—whether intentionally or unintentionally constructed—create and reinforce the belief that MRI exams provide definitive knowledge that is more precise than information provided by other methods.

In analyzing these narratives, I attend not only to those discourses most visible but also to processes rendered invisible, showing how dominant accounts "black box" crucial decisions made by technologists and the interpretive work of radiologists and referring physicians.[1] Each of these actions shape the use and quality of MRI exams in medical practice yet are seldom discussed in popular culture narratives.

Examining the relationships that surround and inform the production of medical images demonstrates that MRI scans are highly mediated representations that are influenced by decisions and values during all aspects of the production process. The images do not *reveal* the inner body, but instead *produce* the body, bringing together aspects of physical bodies, technology, and cultural, social, and economic factors in ways that both include and exceed the physical body. Moreover, textual analysis and ethnographic research combined show that current medical practices and policies rely on the invisibility of physicians and technologists' knowledge about and use of MRI. Imaging policies that require only one interpretation of an image or promote the idea that the image alone offers the "truth" about a patient's condition are sustained and maintained through an erasure of everyday work practices.

Popular Narratives about MRI

Medical imaging is a source of fascination for news media and popular science and a common feature in science exhibits at museums and other

---

[1] For a discussion of black-boxing, see Latour (1987).

sites. MRI is often represented in such accounts, and is understood by health care workers, research scientists, and the public as one of the best and most complicated imaging technologies. Popular narratives construct a singular understanding of MRI images—one that represents them as authoritative knowledge—while simultaneously downplaying other ways of comprehending these artifacts. The many translational processes involved in producing an MRI image, which include human manipulation of the technology, sociotechnical transformations of the data from numerical to pictorial form, and human interpretation of the image, are seldom discussed. In these narratives, MRI exams exist independently of human actions and institutional relations.

Three tropes are recurrently used in news media and popular culture to discuss MRI examinations, and their combined effect imbues the exams with an aura of authority. Tropes, as figurative speech, veer language away from literal meaning and convey layers of ideas through metaphor, synecdoche, and other rhetorical techniques. They carry emotional and symbolic weight as they can transform an object into something more than the thing itself. While all language is tropic, it is not always recognized as such. The point here is not to suggest that technology and science can be spoken about without figurative language, but to highlight the specific metaphors in play. While people's self-consciousness about the language as figurative varies, the repetition of these ideas across multiple sites has important ideological effects. Their repetition shores up the authority of the image and reinforces current imaging policies in the United States.

The Image as Transparent Knowledge

The first trope positions the anatomical picture as interchangeable with the part of the body being scanned instead of a construction of it. This narrative practice assumes that there is an a priori body that exists outside of human mediation and that MRI provides direct access to this material. Here both language and text as well as human and nonhuman interaction are effaced as the "reality" of a transparent body emerges. Discussion of the many layers of human and machine mediation required to create and use MRI exams is typically absent or, if mentioned at all, is addressed in a way that supports the ideal of transparency.

The cultural construction of authoritative knowledge from a transparent body enrolls multiple technologies, media narratives, and cultural ideals. Media studies scholar José van Dijck (2005, 15) traces the ideal of what she calls "corporeal transparency" in an array of medical visualization techniques ranging from operation films to digital cadavers. She finds that in its contemporary form, transparency is linked to other cultural ideals such as perfectibility and malleability and is considered desirable because it allows the body to be manipulated and perfected. Medicine and media come together via health care professionals' interest in promoting cutting-edge techniques and reporters' hunt for new stories to present the ideal of corporeal transparency for consumption among the general public.

The rhetoric of transparency is not limited to representations of medical technologies; it is also found in discussions about discoveries in laboratories and other areas of scientific inquiry (see, e.g., Haraway 1997; Shapin and Schaffer 1985; Traweek 1992). The idea that nature can be known without human mediation and that scientists witness and thus reveal the natural world runs deep in cultural narratives. Appealing to a desire to fully know (and thus control) the world, such an understanding simultaneously erases the many institutional contexts and human actions that coproduce and mediate knowledge. Scholars working at the nexus of science and technology studies and disciplines such as sociology and anthropology research the sociality of scientific knowledge production. Such work shows how scientific knowledge is simultaneously valuable and mediated, and how it produces identities and politics that require critical examination.

The presentation of anatomical MRI images as transparent windows into the body is omnipresent in journalism and print media. "Supersharp scanning machines are giving doctors a clear new window into the brains of stroke victims, revealing strokes that are missed three-quarters of the time by older scanners," writes one reporter (Haney 2000, 29) in a discussion on a new use for MRI. "The device is a kind of souped-up MRI machine that can pinpoint spots of dying tissue deep within the brain during the first hours of a stroke." In this passage, one can see deep into the body through the clear window of MRI and pinpoint things previously unknowable. *Time* magazine journalists Claudia Wallis and Kristina Dell report that Dr. Jay Giedd "has devoted the past 13 years to peering inside the heads of 1,800 kids and teenagers using high-powered magnetic resonance imaging [MRI]. For each volunteer, he creates a unique photo album, taking MRI snapshots every two years and building a record as the brain morphs and grows" (Wallis and Dell 2004, 56). The differences between the MRI exam and the body part being imaged are not mentioned. In this trope, they are one.

The assumption that MRI examinations produce transparency is not only repeated throughout the popular press, but is constructed in academic science texts written for a popular audience as well (see, e.g., Kevles 1997; Wobarst 1999). Anthony Wobarst's (1999, 19) introduction to medical imaging text illustrates this pattern when he writes, "MRI not only reveals the structural details of the various organs, as does CT, but it also provides information on their physiological status and pathologies." Wobarst's use of the words "reveals" and "provides" stresses the similarity between the image and the body part under scrutiny. Possible differences between the two are not mentioned. Historian Bettyann Kevles (1997, 197) relays a similar understanding of the technology when she writes, "MRI is another level of vision, exposing the workings of the most hidden, vital—and soft—organs, the brain and the heart. MRI has shifted our sense of transparency so that we can see those structures whose form and function had previously been the domain of poets and philosophers." Such narratives collapse distinctions between the flesh and the image; the image becomes interchangeable with instead of a construction of the real.

The idea that the body is interchangeable with the image is constructed in part through the use of visual metaphors. In the examples discussed above, a visualization vortex is created as MRI is said to peer, to provide a window, to reveal, and to create a new level of vision. Such visual references draw on broader cultural ideas that privilege sight as a source of knowledge.[2] Sayings like "seeing is believing" and the use of words such as illuminate, illustrate, and inspect to talk about knowledge claims demonstrate the link between sight and evidence in English. Words no longer associated with sight also have visual roots. *Demonstrate*, for example, is derived from the Latin *monstrare*, to show, and *survey* comes from the Middle French *surveeir*, to look over (from *sur-* + *veeir*, to see), and the Latin *supervide*, to oversee.

Mechanically produced pictures have high status as evidence within the realm of sight, and are often thought to provide an unmediated slice of the world. This belief, or what visual culture scholars Marita Sturken and Lisa Cartwright (2001, 17) call "the myth of photographic truth," emphasizes the truth-value of pictures created through mechanical means. MRI exams, which combine technology and the visual, gain authority from this assumption. The link between photographs and anatomical images can be explicit, as in the *Time* magazine article that called MRI examinations "snapshots" that make a "photo album."[3] Such analogies connect the image to family and documentation; they do not connect it to art photography—a visual medium more likely to be understood as fiction. Or, it can be implicit—a cultural code that shapes the meaning attached to

---

[2] Literature that examines the links between sight and knowledge include Berger (1973), Bryson (1994), Jay (1994), Mirzoeff (1998), and Sontag (1990).

[3] Tal Golan (1998) and Bernike Pasveer (1989) demonstrate how the ties between photography and medical images were clearly articulated in the late nineteenth and early twentieth centuries. X-rays were known as "the new photography," and x-ray production was considered a specialty within the field of photography.

a technology made to act through visual metaphors. While scholars have shown that the interpretation of image content is a learned activity (see, e.g., Lynch 1985b; Goodwin 1994, 1995; Prasad 2005b) and that the meaning of images as accurate records of the real is contested (see, e.g., Berger 1973; Dumit 1999; Sontag 1990), the myth of photographic truth continues to be a powerful cultural belief.

The use of technology, as suggested by Sturkin and Cartwright's emphasis on *machine-produced* pictures, is crucial to perceptions of MRI scans as unmediated slices of the body. In an analysis of how definitions of objectivity change over time, Lorraine Daston and Peter Galison (1992, 98) demonstrate that since the late nineteenth century objectivity has been "tied to a relentless search to replace individual volition and discretion in depiction by the invariable routines of mechanical reproduction." Believed to be precise and indefatigable, machines are highly valued in knowledge production. In contrast, the human, positioned as fallible and biased, is transformed into a suspicious figure. The attribution of precision to mechanical reproduction produces a halo of certainty around machine-produced information; numbers, graphs, and anatomical pictures all benefit from this shared belief.

In the case of MRI, its authority is further strengthened by its position in technological hierarchies. Physicians, policy makers, and the press all consider it to be one of the best visualization technologies available. Its perceived status comes in part from its expense (a state-of-the-art machine costs between 1.5 and 2 million dollars, in contrast to a new ultrasound machine which costs between 500,000 and 600,000 dollars), and its complexity. While x-ray, CT, ultrasound, and MRI each have particular clinical situations in which each is the best possible technique, this fact is forgotten when MRI is positioned as the gold standard. Its elite position adds yet more "machineness" to its social identity and thus adds more "precision" to the exactness already attributed to mechanical reproduction. That is, if machines are thought to be reliable producers of knowledge, then the ones at the apex of technohierarchies must be the most precise.

In addition to appealing to cultural beliefs about visualization and mechanical reproduction, the transparency ascribed to MRI is given a magical aspect through use of the word "reveal." Present in two of the examples discussed above, *reveal, from the* Latin *revelare,* meaning "to pull away the veil," is often used to describe the actions of an image. It connotes the veracity associated with sight. However, it also has an otherworldly connotation. The *Oxford English Dictionary* (1989) defines *reveal* as "to disclose, or make known in a supernatural manner" and revelation, a related word, as "the disclosure or communication of knowledge to man by a divine or supernatural agency" (811). Both words are often used in the context of Christianity and in discussions of magic and magicians. Even if reporters and science writers do not use the otherworldly meaning of the word, this meaning can infuse contemporary discourse and imbue the act of looking with a sense of transcendence.

Assertions about the images' ability to produce transparency, whether created through the use of visual, technological, or transcendent metaphors, are often linked to claims about positive health outcomes. Wobarst's book on imaging technologies exemplifies this pattern when he discusses an imaginary case study wherein a patient's ruptured disk is revealed and thus cured through the technology's use. Taking care to distinguish among different images, Wobarst (1999, 167) notes that one picture "shows clearly the rupture (herniation) of one disk" while another "provides precise delineation of the herniation." Continuing with the patient scenario, he concludes, "A week after the MRI scans, Mr. Herndon returned to the operating room to have the damaged disk removed, along with the disk jelly that was pressing on the nerve, and the pain subsided over the next few weeks. He was back on his feet after four days of bed rest, but he was ordered to be extremely gentle with himself for several months" (Wobarst 1999, 167). Here, the scans provide the correct diagnosis—one that leads to the appropriate treatment and the restoration of agility, as well as permission to lead a gentle way of life. Indeed, the book title itself—*Looking Within: How X-ray, CT, MRI, Ultrasound, and Other Medical Images Are Created and How They Help Save Lives*—conveys the idea, to say the least, that imaging use is crucial to the restoration of health.

Wobarst's imaginary patient scenario is not unusual. Popular narratives often associate MRI use with remarkable changes in health outcomes—ones that lead to appropriate medical interventions and result in cures without complications. Scenarios in which a patient has an MRI exam and discovers that his or her disease is too advanced for surgery are not discussed. Nor are cases mentioned that show a patient learning that he or she has an injury and the cure is simply rest. Such examples could be considered successful because the knowledge provided by the technology allowed people to make more informed decisions about their lives.

In all, narratives about MRI examinations are saturated with the notions that they represent unmediated access to a body that exists outside of language and human actions and that they provide definitive answers about a person's physical condition. Through such cultural work, MRI—a thing—now stands for more than itself. No longer simply a machine or an image, it symbolizes unmediated access to the body and is perceived as crucial to the restoration of one's well-being.

MRI as Progress

The second trope found in popular narratives compares MRI scans with the clinical exam and other less expensive technologies. In doing so, the idea that MRI exams represent neutral knowledge that renders the body transparent is further strengthened. Clinical exams and patient histories are always positioned as subjective and inaccurate sources of knowledge, while the MRI or medical image represents a better, more objective, neutral technique.

An article about medical imaging in *FDA Consumer* illustrates this rhetorical practice. Tamar Nordenberg (1999, 12), the author of the article, concludes her discussion of medical imaging with the following passage:

> Wanda Diak's ovarian cancer has not been evident for almost three years. During her follow-up exams, she says, her doctor sometimes taps on her stomach to check for signs of reoccurrence. The method seemed primitive to Diak, but her doctor pointed out that before CT scans and other imaging, different sounds were all doctors had to clue them in to an abnormality. "I think about someone tapping on your stomach rather than having this image that essentially slices you in half so you can see inside," Diak says. "It's like the caveman to the year 2000."

Nordenberg's narrative contrasts medical imaging with the physical exam, suggesting that imaging is superior to other ways of knowing the body. The use of the phrase "different sounds were all doctors had" implies that the knowledge obtained by the physical exam is not as valuable as that provided by medical imaging. The belief is further enforced by the labeling of the physical exam as "primitive"; it is thought to come from the time of "cavemen." In contrast, medical images are linked to the year 2000, which positions them as part of modernity or progress.

The use of comparison—which is crucial to the positioning of MRI images as unbiased and the producer of certainty—is relied on in many cultural sites. An exhibit at Epcot cosponsored by the Radiological Society of North America (RSNA) and Disney, for example, illustrates this type of narrative strategy. The video that featured MRI—called "an adventure" by the Disney Imagineers—provides an important example of how MRI exams get positioned as true and objective while the clinical exam and other "low-tech" procedures often get labeled as misleading and subjective.

The Epcot "adventure" begins with a voice-over that says, "Let's let the MRI tell the story. With it we've eliminated guesswork from diagnosis."

After this statement, the film moves to an enactment of a short discussion between an Olympic athlete and her doctor. In the fictional interaction, the athlete expresses concern and anxiety about her ability to compete in the upcoming events. She had injured her ankle and was unsure about the extent of the damage. The physician looks at the MRI exam to answer the athlete's questions. After studying the images, the doctor declares that the ankle injury is not a problem. As the video concludes, it shows the athlete (now cured) successfully competing in an Olympic event.

The video, like the previous example, illustrates MRI's positioning in the public realm as objective and as the primary producer of knowledge, not only of a patient's condition but also of one's possibilities. Other techniques, such as the patient history and the physical exam, are relegated to the margins as potential, yet less accurate, forms of knowledge. The opening narrative makes this clear: "With [MRI] we have eliminated the guess-work from diagnosis." This statement positions MRI as true, accurate knowledge and other techniques as subjective interpretation. The video includes no reference to the use of the patient's history or clinical evaluation as a way to diagnose the ankle problem. Instead, viewers are led to believe that MRI scans provide the answer and reduce the risk of wrong diagnosis, thus enhancing a person's ability to be in control and compete in life's challenges.[4]

This way of framing MRI exams is repeated throughout popular culture and mass media narratives. The use of comparison bolsters the view that MRI provides a superior form of knowledge—one that is objective and complete. It also reinforces the notion that use of MRI technology removes subjectivity from the process of diagnosis.

MRI as Agent

The third rhetorical strategy used to discuss MRI positions both the images and the technology as actors. Across cultural narratives, MRI is given

---

[4] Few popular representations of MRI challenge the idea that the image is superior to the clinical exam. Examples include the August 8, 2000, episode of the sitcom *Becker*. In this show, the main character, Dr. Becker, uses a stethoscope to diagnose a patient's illness. An MRI exam is then ordered to corroborate the diagnosis. Here, MRI is portrayed as a technique that is used in conjunction with others; it is not presented as "better than" than the stethoscope or the clinical exam. An episode of *Providence*, another TV show that features a physician, also challenged conventional technological hierarchies. In the September 8, 2000, episode, a neurologist insists on the importance of the patient history. Although he has the information provided by the MRI exam, he notes that "That's the problem with a patient in a coma. You are missing your star witness." These examples challenge the view that MRI is superior to the clinical exam, and remain rare in popular culture in the United States.

an almost magical power. The distinction between machine and image is often blurred as MRI confirms, reveals, and finds the presence of disease and injuries. An article about a young woman's struggle with brain cancer exemplifies this approach when the reporter writes, "MRI scans found cancer in her brain" (Parlette 2005, E1). Or, as Kevles (1997, 175) writes when discussing the 1991 trial about the police beating of Rodney King, "The MRI showed the jury where cerebral spinal fluid had leaked through multiple skull fractures (seen on accompanying CT images) into King's right maxillary sinus." In these and other examples, the image/machine is positioned as an actor—one that is capable of finding or showing weighty knowledge about the body.

The repetition of this rhetorical practice across popular narratives positions MRI as an actor—one who creates authoritative knowledge and provides access to unseen parts of the body. As Donna Haraway and Bruno Latour have argued, humans are *not* the only ones represented as actors in discussions about science and technology. Nonhumans are ascribed agency in narratives as well. Transformed into agents, these nonhuman actors are then able to advance different positions (Haraway 1997, 143; Latour 1993, 38–40).[5] These positions can represent any political goal—there is no one way to make nonhumans act. For example, a technoscience agent such as the Oncomouse (a genetically modified laboratory mouse designed to develop cancer) can be used to promote animal rights or challenge it.

In this case, the positioning of MRI as an actor further advances the idea that the image provides neutral knowledge. It reinforces the notion that the machine and the images produced by it create and reveal the truth about a person's body. It encourages the idea that human values and social contexts do not "taint" this form of information about health and illness. The repetition of the trope (coupled with the neglect of other stories about the technology and the image) makes it harder to imagine if, how, where, and when human decisions and institutional priorities shape the quality of these examinations.

These three ways of talking about MRI examinations and technology were common across a diverse set of texts in the public realm. These tropes were also utilized by members of the medical community during my fieldwork

[5] Haraway (2003) takes this argument a step further by positioning nonhumans as actors in the social world. She suggests that we should theorize nonhumans as subjects; let ourselves be affected by nonhuman actors; and include their interests in evaluations of new technoscientific practices.

and interviews. These narratives, however, were not the only ones used by physicians and technologists. Physicians and technologists are flexible discursive actors who occupy multiple social worlds. These locations—which include various local cultures within the clinic and the broader social milieu—allow physicians and technologists to speak about the image and the technology in a variety of ways.[6]

Medical Narratives about MRI

In my research, radiologists, technologists, and referring physicians used multiple narratives to discuss MRI. The three tropes observed in popular culture and media accounts were one set of discursive strategies mobilized by physicians and technologists to discuss MRI with colleagues, patients, and observers such as myself. While the physicians and technologists understood—through their work practices and training—that the image does not render the body transparent, they often used popular rhetorical practices to articulate observations about MRI exams in everyday conversations with each other and patients.

First, physicians and technologists at the research sites used narratives that conflated the anatomical image with the body. One physician stated, for example, "MRI is really the same as the anatomy labs. You can look at the anatomy perfectly, see everything." Another explained, "Now with MRI you are going to be seeing the heart in real time. You are going to be seeing the lungs in real time. You are going to be marching through the body with MRI." These quotes are representative of a general trend that I found among the interviews. As in the public discourse, MRI scans were discussed in a way that suggests these exams provide unmediated access to the truth of the body. The common use of words such as *seeing* and *look* highlight the visual component of MRI exams. In this way, seeing becomes linked to transparency, and the virtual becomes the real.

These same medical professionals also utilized the comparison of MRI scans to other techniques to bolster the view that medical images represent objective knowledge. One radiologist noted, for example, "Physical exams are guesses as to what is going on. The imaging is really key." Another doctor stated, "Using MRI, one can easily look and see that there is a disc [problem in the back]. It's all very cut and dried. It's not like, 'Oh well. I can do an examination on you and [tell you that] you have some sort of

---

[6] For an excellent discussion of the heterogeneity of medical practice and the multiple identities and narratives used by medical actors, see Berg and Mol (1998).

lower back pain. We don't know exactly what's causing it. It's probably a disc.'" In these narratives, the contrast between MRI and other techniques is used to emphasize the authority of medical images. The MRI exam is considered to be "very cut and dried"; it is the "key" that leads to certainty and knowledge.

The belief that MRI exams produce certainty further promotes the idea that the ambiguity of disease and diagnosis can be eliminated. Some of the physicians I interviewed articulated the idea that MRI scans can minimize the uncertainty of the diagnostic process. One radiologist stated, for example, "MR is something very nice to learn, something clean. It is usually straightforward to come up with a diagnosis." This radiologist's use of the words "clean" and "straightforward" suggest that he believes that the images are able to reduce the complexity of disease into a clearly defined entity. Other physicians articulated this idea as well. One noted, "One nice thing about the radiology image is that it's all there. I often feel sorry for some of my clinical colleagues, the internists particularly, who have to listen for a long, long time to decide that there isn't anything that this patient has that they can do anything about. I personally found it kind of frustrating to have to listen to sixty minutes of dissertation of a patient's symptoms which don't add up to disease." In this account the image has "it all"; it eliminates the confusion, or perhaps messiness, of listening to patients as well as the problem of not being able to come up with a diagnosis.

Finally, the physicians and technologists also employed language practices that position MRI technology and the images produced by it as agents. This practice was not as common in my fieldwork and interviews as it was in the mass media accounts, but it did occur. A radiologist illustrated this practice when he explained, "It was MRI that diagnosed that problem. MRI has told me that the patient has had strokes, but I don't know what caused it." Another radiologist noted, "It [MRI] shows you so much . . . It's just so fantastic. It shows you everything you have to see." Or, as one physician stated, "Here is an equipment which allows you to know a lot and peeps into your body and has the ability even to look at functions and things like that." In this way, the technology is rhetorically positioned as an actor—one who talks and peeps.

In all, the three tropes were an integral component of language practices in imaging units. The use of the tropes provides a way to think about the complex relations among medical professionals, culture, and technology. First, the use of all three tropes demonstrates how medicine is a social practice that simultaneously is influenced by and influences cultural narratives about identity, knowledge, and health.[7] Radiologists, technologists, and referring physicians—as actors in a broader cultural milieu—use available interpretations and frames to explain the images and technology. Demonstrating the force of culture, they use this language as a convenient shorthand even though they know through work practices that such statements do not fully capture the relations between the image and the body nor how the technology is used in health care. In turn, the physicians and technologists' use of the narrative techniques reinforces the use of them in other social fields such as the media and popular culture. While it has little effect if a few individuals use common narratives, the accumulation of their use across medicine and popular culture reinforces the idea that the image is superior to other forms of knowledge. Embedded in culture, science simultaneously produces it.

Second, the decision to use these tropes is further bolstered by the location of these particular physicians and technologists in clinical medical practice. As noted in chapter 2, there are multiple ways to discuss medical images of the brain; professional contexts support the choice of particular rhetorical practices over others. For example, research scientists use numerical metaphors to discuss brain images, whereas clinical radiologists rely on pictorial language to describe the same type of scans (Beaulieu 2002). The radiologists, referring physicians, and technologists interviewed and observed for this project all practice in clinical medicine. The use of pictorial language to describe anatomical images is supported by this context as radiologists, physicians, and patients primarily work with the visual component of the exam. The numerical values are not directly pertinent to their work. In addition, radiologists are trained to interpret minute visual details and are part of a profession that defines itself as authorities on visualization. The combination of the local culture of clinical medicine and the professional culture of radiology reinforces physicians and technologists' tendency to embrace the tropes discussed above as they emphasize the visuality of MRI exams.

Finally, the physicians and technologists' use of the third trope—MRI as agent—demonstrates the complex relations humans have with machines and other beings. Many people imagine the regularly encountered others in their lives—be they animals or machines—in an anthropomorphic manner. Personification suggests the close relation between health

---

[7] Social science research that examines how physicians and scientists are simultaneously informed by and produce culture include Clarke et al. (2003), Guillemin and Holmstrom (1999), Martin (1987), Martin (1995), and Oudshoorn (1994).

care professionals and the machine itself, and can be read as a sign of deep connection.

The use of the trope also legitimizes the MRI exam as statements such as "the machine told me" circulate in a context that positions mechanical reproduction as reliable and precise. As noted earlier, mechanical reproduction is thought to create trustworthy knowledge, whereas human actors are perceived as subjective and fallible. "Western medicine is dominated by a single imperative—the quest for machinelike perfection in the delivery of care," writes surgeon Atul Gawande (2002, 37–38). "When I am in the operating room, the highest praise I can receive from my fellow surgeons is 'You're a machine, Gawande.' " In a framework that links perfection and precision to mechanical reproduction, to be considered highly skilled is to be labeled a machine. Statements like "I interpreted the image and found . . ." bring the potentially unreliable human being back into the knowledge-making process—an unsettling move in a symbolic milieu that privileges machines as consistent and exact.

In an emotionally charged climate such as health care, the transference of action from human to machine not only bolsters the perceived reliability of the information but also shifts responsibility for it from human to technology. While the law and professional ethics require physicians and technologists to take responsibility for their work, and many do, accountability is not clearly assigned when the machine is designated as an actor. The rhetorical transfer of responsibility from human to machine has two main effects. First, it makes it easier for health care professionals to negotiate interpersonal encounters; that is, if the machine is perceived as the producer of knowledge, then the physician does not have to explain his or her decisions about how to interpret it. Second, the reassignment of accountability allows physicians and technologists to have psychological distance from the gravity of their work. Health care professionals work with humans at their most vulnerable, and their decisions can have significant effects in a patient's quality of life. Positioning the MRI as agent temporarily shifts responsibility from human to machine and distances physicians and technologists from the human implications and consequences of their decisions as they create and interpret anatomical images.

The epistemological effects of the continual use of all three tropes by physicians, technologists, journalists, and popular science writers are significant. The use of the tropes shores up the authority of images as an objective source of knowledge that is crucial to the production of definitions of health and illness. These narratives construct one possible way to understand MRI exams: as providing unmediated access to the physical body, a body that can be known and that exists outside of human relations.

Further, they also produce the notion that these exams are authoritative and that they represent progress.

Physicians and technologists are flexible discursive actors, however, who employ a range of narratives to discuss both the image and the technology. Although they used the three tropes to talk about MRI in general, physicians and technologists also used narratives that highlighted how the image is mediated by human decisions and differs from the body in the machine. These accounts—which were articulated when the physicians and technologists explained their work practices or when they described what they perceived of as errors or intrusions in the image—emphasize the instability of MRI and provide an avenue for the critique of popular discourses.

Invisible Practices: The Social Production of MRI Exams

An MRI scan—like all representations—is a constructed artifact.[8] Despite common narratives that position these exams as existing outside of social relations, there are many sites in their production, interpretation, and use that transform them from conveyers of objective, authoritative knowledge into socially situated objects that construct the body in complicated ways. The following sections discuss three sites—the production of the exams, the transformation of the image into a written report, and the use of the scans and the written report by referring physicians—in detail to illustrate how MRI exams produce a "located, embodied, and contingent" truth that merges bodies, machines, and work practices to constitute a particular body in medical practice and social life (Haraway 1997, 230).[9]

This discussion draws on extensive analysis of referring physicians, radiologists, and technologists' tacit knowledge. Tacit knowledge refers to knowledge acquired through the *doing* of science (Collins 1974, 2001).[10] While this knowledge can be articulated, it seldom is. Instead, it remains a form of tacit knowledge that is crucial to the practice of scientific work. The production and use of MRI images also involves the employment of knowledge that is accumulated through working with the technology, and, while an integral component of everyday work practices, is normally unarticulated. Indeed, it is difficult, if not impossible, to fully formulate. Discussion

---

[8] Science and technology studies on the production and use of representations in science include Lynch and Woolgar (1990) and Yoxen (1987).

[9] For an extended discussion of situated knowledge, see Haraway (1988).

[10] For further discussion of Harry Collins's development and use of *tacit knowledge*, see Collins and Kusch (1998).

of physicians and technologists' tacit knowledge creates an understanding of the instability of MRI exams, countering the definitiveness and certainty constructed by common rhetorical practices.

The language used by physicians and technologists to describe variation in and problems with the content and interpretation of images will also be used to analyze the translation processes involved in the production and use of MRI exams. The processes through which scientists translate knowledge into narrative discussions for other actors' understanding is central to scientific work (Latour 1987). Drawing on Michael Lynch's (1985a) analysis of shop talk in a research laboratory, I show how the presence of and talk about artifacts—while understood by medical professionals as distortions of the real—challenge the view that images "reveal" the body. Artifacts provide a visible symbol of the always occurring interpretation work of medical science, illustrating how the real can be constructed only through action and practice. Similarly, discussions about overinterpretation, underdiagnosis, old friends, and unidentified bright objects (UBOs)—while positioned as error or intrusion by medical actors—signal how the creation and use of images are embedded in social relations and cannot exist outside these networks.

The turn to a discussion of image production and use demonstrates the importance of methods such as ethnomethodology and ethnography, which provide access to the multiple discourses and the tacit knowledge used by physicians and technologists as they translate their work practices. While social scientists are not ventriloquists who speak for these medical actors or reveal these social spaces, use of ethnographic methods produces situated analyses of work practices, which, in the case of MRI, complicates popular accounts that suggest anatomical images provide transparent knowledge about the body and health.

Bodies and Machines: Technologists Construct Images

Technologists work directly with both the patient and the machine, and they have an important role in constructing MRI scans. During examinations, technologists assist patients into machines. After carefully positioning a patient, the technologist leaves the examination room and enters another room where the computer screen and terminal are located. Sitting at the computer screen, the technologist uses computer programs to decide the width of a particular picture, the total amount of the area being scanned, the resolution of a particular image, and other technical decisions. Like filmmakers or photographers, technologists have to frame the area that will be included in each picture. These decisions, or parameters, create the images, shaping the content in specific and significant ways.

The effects of a particular parameter—slice thickness—illustrate this point. To create an MRI exam, technologists have to divide the area of the body being imaged into sections and decide the width or thickness of these sections. These decisions change the content of each resulting image produced. With MRI technology, large, thick slices have less spatial resolution than smaller, thin ones. The use of wide slices can therefore erase small lesions or pathologies that might have shown up in images made from thinner segments. These choices therefore hold consequence for what the image looks like.

There are many other choices, such as field of view and number of slices, that support the construction of each anatomical picture. Technologists have to decide values for a range of parameters—each of which will influence what is made to appear and disappear in an image. In my research, technologists—in response to questions about their actions at the computer keyboard and screen—explained how their decisions about parameter values shaped the content of an image. One technologist noted, "It's easy to tweak the parameters to make something that's not there. You can also hide lesions. If you knew where a lesion was and you pointed it out to me, I could make it so that the lesion can be in the gap. And you could go through the liver or the brain and you would never see it." Another technologist reinforced this view, noting that MRI exams are all "smoke and mirrors."

The body is already in a process of translation and interpretation. Decisions made by technologists constitute, via productions and erasures, pathology and its absence in each given image. These visible symbols of "disease" or "health" may have no physical referent in the body being scanned. Examining medical practice and understanding the use of tacit knowledge makes this clear. The technologists' knowledge of how they manipulate image content demonstrates how MRI scans do not provide a transparent "window" into the inner body but instead *produce* the body.

Another moment in the production process—the creation and presence of artifacts—also troubles language practices that equate the image with transparency. *Artifacts* are forms or shapes that appear in an image, and they have many causes. In an MRI image they can appear as black spots, white spots, wavy lines, or create doubles of the area of the body under scrutiny. Artifacts are considered *effects* of the technology by technologists and radiologists, and they are not perceived as useful for understanding the condition of a particular body. However, as noted earlier, Michael Lynch's (1985a, 82–84) research shows how the presence of and reference to artifacts undermines the claim that scientific representations "discover" the

natural world. The presence of artifacts reinscribes the sociotechnical relations that produce the image, signaling how the real can be known only
through social practices.

Cross talk is one artifact of many that can be generated during the production of an exam. This particular artifact—which appears as tiny white
dots in the image—occurs when technologists or radiologists place the sections of the body being measured too close together. One technologist described this phenomenon when she noted, "If you slice sequentially, which
is how most MRI exams are done, and you have really thin slices, the slices
kind of overlap, so there's excitation [of hydrogen protons] above and
below, and that creates the misinformation we call cross talk. You get these
little white dots [in the image] and you're like, 'What the hell is that?' "

"What the hell is that?" may be the response to the identification of artifacts in an image, but artifacts can also be interpreted as anatomy. The
interpretation of artifacts as the body or distortion occurs in the next
stage of production: the translation of the image into words.

Written Reports: Physicians "Read" the Image

After an MRI examination, the images created are sent to a physician who
produces a written report that translates the content of the images into
words. Physicians—through this act of interpretation—produce the presence of health or illness in particular images and by extension in particular patients. Usually the physicians who "read" or interpret MRI exams are
radiologists. Diagnostic radiologists complete a bachelor's degree, a medical doctor (MD) or a doctor of osteopathy's (DO) degree, and a four-year
residency in radiology with the aim of specializing in the interpretation of
visual depictions of anatomy. Legally, however, any MD or DO is allowed
to interpret medical images. Reading images is similar, in terms of process, to other methods of diagnosis. The doctor must analyze the image
within the context of a patient's history, the clinical examination, and
other test results.

Most imaging sites employ one radiologist who primarily works on his
or her own. This doctor is responsible for interpreting the exams produced by a particular facility. Large hospitals provide an exception to this
practice; these institutions hire multiple radiologists who work similar
hours. A challenging case may lead a radiologist to consult others in his or
her unit. For the most part, though, these physicians labor alone, translating visual anatomy into written text day in and day out.

Image interpretation work is a socially situated activity; it is not the
transparent process constructed by dominant accounts. Radiologists have

to learn—through interaction with other physicians and machines—to "see" cross talk and other artifacts as well as variations in spacing, light, and human anatomy in MRI scans. They discipline and train their sight overtime to code and highlight aspects of the image content.[11]

This disciplining is, of course, a continual process that is enacted each time a physician interprets an image. As repetitive actions, such activities are open to divergent interpretations and contestation from individuals using the same perceptual framework. Indeed, research shows that controversy and discrepancy are common in radiologists' interpretation practices (see, e.g., Beam, Layde, and Sullivan 1996; Laming and Warren 2000; Reiser 1978). The vision of radiologists is thus simultaneously disciplined, ordered, and open to divergent interpretations.

Medical workers have developed language to discuss discrepancies in interpretation. Two common terms used to describe sources of error are underdiagnosis and overinterpretation. Both "problems" occur regularly in medical practice, and they are integral components of interpretation work. The occurrence of and discussion about interpretation troubles—as with artifacts—demonstrate how the knowledge produced through the use of medical images is continually influenced by human actions and decisions. The always occurring interpretation work, in other words, is made visible in discursive practices when problems arise.

Underdiagnosis is a term used by medical professionals to describe situations in which the radiologist interprets the anatomy in the image as normal, but other physicians identify pathology in the same image. All radiologists at times underdiagnose the content of images. As one radiologist explained, "You hope that you see everything, but that isn't the case. There have been studies that suggest that radiologists may miss 35 percent of the findings on any given image."

Another interpretation practice that is discussed by physicians and medical practitioners is overinterpretation. *Overinterpretation* describes instances in which a radiologist labels the anatomy in the image "abnormal," but the information produced through a second interpretation of the same image, or through use of other techniques, such as the patient history, blood tests, or surgery, suggest that the anatomy in the image is "normal" for that patient. This occurs in part because radiologists have to continually decide whether the content of an image represents stable

[11] The processes and interactions that train and discipline radiologists' sight over time deserve further analysis. In-depth study of how radiologists learn to "see" or "read" images would provide insight into how sight is itself a social practice that is learned through interaction with people and machines (Prasad 2005a, 2005b).

anatomy, disease, or artifact. This interpretation work is especially challenging because there is a wide range of anatomical details that are considered "healthy" for potential patients and because artifacts often resemble the visible presentation of disease.

Unidentified Bright Objects (UBOs) and Old Friends

Bodies exhibit a variety of anatomical details in MRI scans. Although the majority of patients have similar anatomical features in an image, there is a significant group that falls outside of these normative patterns. Physicians who work with MRI have developed language to identify this diversity. Many of the physicians I interviewed, for instance, discussed the appearance of UBOs, or "unidentified bright objects." As one physician explained, "You can find things [in the image] that are difficult to interpret. Like what people call UBOs." Another physician commented, "You must have heard of UBOs, or unidentified bright objects. Patients will see the radiology report and say, 'Well, what does that mean?' I say, 'It probably doesn't mean anything. Maybe it is because you hit your head some time ten years ago or you have a migraine or whatever.' "

Another physician referred to UBOs, but he called these bright objects "old friends." He stated, "A favorite line of one of my own professors back when I was a resident, was 'Well, I don't know what it is but I know that it's not important. It's an old friend.' " This physician further explained that "old friends" appear in images because there is variation among bodies. He noted, "Some of these old friends are simply anatomic variations from person to person. We all have different noses, different eye color, and different looking hair. You know that all those hairs and noses are normal, but they all look different. There are variations in the brain as well. When you see these variations day after day, if you are not sure what they are, you work them up, and gradually they become old friends."

When translating an image into text, radiologists have to decide whether to label the anatomy in the image an "UBO" or "disease." Radiologists—as part of this interpretation process—at times translate parts of the image as abnormal when they might be UBOs for that particular person. As one physician explained, "If I were to take a hundred outwardly normal people and take MRIs of their brains, maybe twenty people are going to have something that is going to be read out by a very good radiologist as not quite normal." In this instance "not quite normal" implies that it will be interpreted as "disease." In these cases, the patient with the supposed "disease" may undergo more tests to determine if there is really a problem or, in the worst-case scenario, endure treatments for this supposed condition.

Radiologists may also construct the presence of disease by labeling arti-facts in an image "pathology." Radiologists—when faced with particular shapes in an image—have to decide whether they represent anatomy or an artifact. This interpretive work becomes even more challenging when arti-facts look the same as the visible presentation of pathology. For example, the *cross talk* artifact discussed earlier can mimic the anatomical forms as-sociated with multiple sclerosis. Other artifacts also mirror the appear-ance of disease as well.

Radiologists—through the interpretation process—thus can and do in-terpret artifacts as disease. One physician I interviewed described a case in which a patient was diagnosed with a tumor that was later interpreted as an artifact. She stated,

> There was a patient at ———— that was scheduled to have a resection of a pineal tumor. It turned out that it was an artifact from a flow void. The neurosurgeon who scheduled the operation for that same day said, "I just want to make sure that we are looking at the same thing here." He put the film up in front of me. And I said, "We are looking at a flow void in the third ventricle." He said, "Really? That's not a pineal tumor?" I said, "No. That's not a pineal tumor." And he said, "Oh. Good thing I showed it to you."

In this example, the radiologist who initially interpreted the image la-beled the artifact produced by blood flow "a tumor" in her report. The neurosurgeon, however, happened to ask for a second opinion before starting the surgery. The second radiologist convinced the surgeon that the supposed "tumor" was an artifact. This second interpretation was in turn supported by other clinical information, and the patient did not undergo surgery. If the neurosurgeon had not asked for a second view, the patient would have had surgery for a disease he did not have. Al-though this patient was able to avoid this, there are occasions when in-terpretation discrepancies are not noticed and unnecessary treatment occurs.

In addition to these routine problems, one must remember that inter-pretation is work done by people, and, as with all jobs, the quality of per-formance varies. When asked how a patient should evaluate a prospective imaging facility, radiologists and referring physicians explained that it is important to choose sites that have highly skilled radiologists. One radiol-ogist I interviewed, for example, noted, "The accuracy of the MRI exam is heavily dependent on the quality of the radiologists who interpret them." Another physician cautioned, "You have got to try to pick places where the radiologists are going to be good. People don't understand that it's not just about the technology. You can get pictures, but it's the interpretation of those pictures that's key." The radiologists' interpretive work and variability is seldom made visible by commonly used discourses about MRI. Discussion of radiologists' tacit knowledge and narratives about perceived error demonstrates how medical images construct the body; they do not reveal it.

Clinical Practices: MRI and Other Diagnostic Tests

Narratives that suggest MRI exams provide unbiased knowledge, and thus reveal the truth about the health of a person's body, also erase how referring physicians—the doctors who initially order the MRI exams—use medical images in conjunction with other tests to make sense of a person's situation. Referring physicians seldom use solely the information obtained via MRI technology to diagnose a patient. Instead they look at the information provided by an array of methods to create a better understanding of a particular individual's body. Through this iterative process, referring physicians integrate the knowledge obtained by the MRI exam with other information. In practice, MRI findings can and do contradict information obtained via other tests about a patient's condition. There are two ways that this can occur. In the first situation, the information provided by MRI indicates there is no disease, whereas the information provided by other techniques suggests there is disease present. In the second situation, the interpretation of the MRI scans indicates disease, while other clinical findings suggest that there is no disease.

In interviews, referring physicians—when explaining the tacit knowledge acquired and used in their work practices—provided examples of both possible scenarios. Many physicians mentioned, for example, instances in which the MRI exam indicated no disease, while the clinical exam revealed the opposite.[12] One such example is multiple sclerosis (MS).

[12] The clinical or physical exam and the patient history refer to two distinct components of an office visit. An office visit generally begins with a discussion of the patient's understanding of his or her health. After taking a patient's medical history, a clinician (e.g., physician, nurse practitioner) conducts a physical or clinical exam. During the physical exam, the health care professional may visually inspect the body, use palpitation to examine the main organ systems, and conduct other relevant tests. Although the patient history and the physical exam are clearly connected to each other, they are considered two distinct activities within medicine. The distinction between the two activities maintains the boundary between information given by patients and information observed by clinicians—a boundary that is reinforced in other medical categories such as signs (i.e., the clinical manifestations observed by the clinician) and symptoms (i.e., the description of the illness experience by the patient).

MS lesions in the brain can show up as bright or dark patches in an MRI exam, depending on the techniques used. Despite this, there are cases when a patient has all of the clinical findings of multiple sclerosis, yet the MRI scan appears normal. As one neurologist pointed out, "The MRI scan is probably negative up to 25 percent of the time in [MS] cases, so I would usually trust my exam much more than the MRI scan." In this situation, the physician has to rely on other indicators to produce a diagnosis. The MRI findings are misleading and inaccurate; it is the clinical exam that provides the useful information about the patient's condition.

In addition to these types of situations, physicians also have to balance indications of abnormality in MRI scans with the information provided by other techniques such as the clinical exam. Throughout my research, referring physicians discussed the importance of the clinical exam as the knowledge produced by its use helped sort out which information in an MRI scan is relevant. One noted, for example, "Say a patient gets an MRI and it shows a lesion that is of no clinical consequence. Now you are left with doing the backtracking and saying, 'You're neurologically normal. This bright object in your brain is of no significance. It has no correlation with the headache that you have. You just have a headache.'" For this doctor, the clinical exam and other diagnostic tests provide the framework needed to make sense of the information given by MRI. Without other sources of information, physicians and patients might spend a lot of time treating and watching abnormalities in an image that actually reflect stable pathology or a normal feature of that person's body. As one physician explained, "Just because the radiologist saw something doesn't mean that it's relevant."

The Value of Patient Histories and Clinical Exams

Patient histories and clinical exams are also needed to use MRI technology appropriately in diagnostic work. One physician explained, "Say somebody comes into the ER and has arm weakness. Arm weakness can be caused by a stroke in the brain. It can be caused by a disc in the neck. It can also be caused by carpal tunnel syndrome in the wrist and so on. All of these conditions present as arm weakness." Taking a good personal history allows a physician to narrow down the possible causes of the arm weakness. If they neglect to do this, they may well order an MRI examination that is unrelated to the person's symptoms. For example, they may order a scan of the brain when it is actually a neck problem. In this case, a brain image is useless.

The reversal of the typical technological hierarchy between low-tech procedures and MRI examinations was noted by others as well. One technologist explained, "You have leg pain. Radiating pain down your leg. It could be caused by mets [metastasis] in your back, even though it is not your spine that is hurting. So you can have symptoms that are not really related to that area." In this situation, the patient history and physical exam allow physicians to figure out which area of the body to image. Without these tools, physicians would not know which part of the body to scan because pain in a certain location can have multiple causes and be generated by different parts of the body.

The clinical exam and patient history are also needed to narrow down the area to be imaged. One technologist explained, for instance, "MRI is very organ specific. You can't have a patient come in for a screen. We get a lot of doctors that call and say, 'I want an abdomen.' We say, 'Well, what do you want to see?' The doctor says, 'She has abdomen pain.' We say, 'What do you want to see? You can see the liver, you can see the kidney, you can see the adrenal gland, you can see the spleen. But you can't see all of them together. The studies for the liver aren't the same as the ones for the kidney. You need to do different types of MRI studies to see each organ clearly.' " The clinical exam and patient history are thus necessary to narrow down which organs need to be imaged. Without the information provided by the patient and the clinical exam, the technologists and radiologists would not know which organ to choose; the way MRI works does not allow them to capture a whole area of the body in one scan. Instead, individual organs must be singled out.

Institutional Practices and Policies Shape MRI Exam Quality

MRI exams are not equivalent to the inner body; instead they produce the body, drawing together technology, the body, and work practices in complex ways. Anatomical images "etch together" local decisions and priorities, technology, and aspects of the physical body to produce what is perceived as cutting-edge, authoritative knowledge (Grosz 1994). "Etching," as developed by Elizabeth Grosz, emphasizes how representations of the body always include and merge parts of the physical body with political hierarchies and technical practices to produce what counts as the body in social life.[13] In the case of MRI, tropes that suggest these examinations exist outside of the realm of human actions make it harder to understand

[13] In her work, Elizabeth Grosz (1994) primarily focuses on written representations of the body. I extend her notion of etching to analyze another site of knowledge production: anatomical pictures.

and analyze the relationships that exist among bodies, technology, actions in imaging units, and anatomical pictures. They render the local knowledge of those who work with and use MRI technology invisible. The political implications of this erasure become clear when the institutional contexts that shape and influence work practices are examined.

The choices made during the production of MRI exams—about parameters, interpretation, and use—occur within larger social fields that influence them. Institutional practices and health care policies shape the decisions and activities made in imaging units and hospitals, and these regulations and routines vary according to the regional and temporal location of a particular imaging site. Current U.S. regulations and institutional practices produce a particular type of MRI examination—one that emphasizes revenue and efficiency over quality.

There are currently no policies in the United States that mandate standards for slice thickness, field of view, and other parameters that shape the content of images. The Food and Drug Administration (FDA) permits manufacturers to build a wide range of value choices into the machines, and this allows administrators, physicians, and technologists greater flexibility in their decisions about what to include and exclude in images.[14] The lack of stringent standards is particularly important because in the case of MRI, decisions about parameter values are also decisions about the length of time required to produce an exam and the degree of spatial resolution. Technological constraints currently require imaging facilities to choose between shorter scan times and increased visibility of anatomical details.

Slice Thickness

A brief discussion of slice thickness—the parameter discussed earlier—provides an example of what this means in practice. With MRI technology, decisions about slice thickness are also decisions about the level of anatomical detail included in an image *and* the length of exam time; short scan times and increased spatial resolution are mutually exclusive effects of the technique. Images based on wide slices simultaneously take less time to

[14] The Food and Drug Administration [FDA] initially gained jurisdiction over medical devices with the passage of the Food, Drug, and Cosmetic Act in 1938. Their authority, however, was limited to challenging the sale of devices believed to be unsafe and to investigating claims made about effectiveness that were false (Merrill 1994). The FDA's regulatory control over medical devices was expanded and formalized with the passage of the Medical Device Amendments in 1976. The Medical Device Amendments allows the FDA to classify and control medical devices through activities such as premarket approval, review of performance, and review of marketing claims (Munsey 1995). As a medical device, MRI procedures fall under the FDA's purview.

produce and include less anatomical detail than images based on thin slices. Wider slices thus potentially erase small lesions or other important anatomical details that would have been included in thinner ones. This same exam, however, takes less time to produce than one based on thinner slices. The trade-off between time and increased visibility is true for other parameters as well. Through decisions about how much of the body to include in an image, choices about speed and quality are also enacted.

The flexibility of parameter choices suggests that decisions about time and visibility are open to the values and imperatives of local institutional contexts. Both nonprofit and for-profit MRI units in the United States are currently under pressure to increase production and income. Since U.S. health care relies on a fee-for-service system of reimbursement, facilities can increase their profit by increasing the number of examinations performed each day. The combination of the fee-for-service payment system and the pressure to increase revenue creates an environment that encourages administrators to make choices that decrease scan time so that more exams, and thus more income, are produced each day. The lack of formal regulation about parameter standards supports these decisions, allowing the time required to create an exam to take precedence over the quality of spatial resolution. While other institutional priorities such as concern about lawsuits may temper this tendency, the pressure to produce revenue is strong; the prioritizing of time over quality is structured into medical policies and practices.

Interpretation Practices

Institutional contexts and regulations also shape the interpretation work of radiologists. Current policies and practices help produce a particular type of written report—one that varies in quality and is least likely to help patients and medical professionals in their quest for health and knowledge. Three policies in particular shape interpretation practices in U.S. medical care. First, despite awareness of the variability of radiologists' interpretation skills, there are few regulations that require formal review of their work. Most imaging centers are not legally required to review radiologists' reports to see if their findings were supported by other tests and information.[15] Radiologists often instead rely on informal feedback from colleagues to gauge their reading abilities.

[15] An exception to this practice is mammography. The Mammography Quality Standards Act (MQSA) allows federal and state inspectors to review "positive" interpretations of mammograms (i.e., the reports that diagnosed cancer in a particular patient) with other clinical information such as biopsies in order to evaluate a particular facility's interpretation work.

Some institutions do have formal processes of evaluation. At these locations, as one physician explained, "radiologists may take random samplings, maybe 10 percent of the cases, and then read each other's images" to estimate the proficiency of radiologists. Other MRI facilities periodically send out images to a third party who then reviews the images for accuracy. These types of systematic reviews are not required by law. Implementation of formal evaluations of radiologists' reading abilities remains up to the initiative of a particular institution.

Second, most insurance companies reimburse MRI units for one reading fee. This practice occurs even though studies have shown the quality of the interpretation increases significantly if two radiologists interpret each exam (see, e.g., Beam, Layde, and Sullivan 1996; Laming and Warren 2000). Despite these findings, typically only one radiologist is paid to view an exam, and most institutions thus have one radiologist interpret a scan.

Third, there are no federal laws that mandate the interpretation of MRI exams be done by physicians trained in this practice. Although some states such as Rhode Island require minimum training in MRI interpretation, most require simply that a medical doctor must produce the official interpretation of an image. In the majority of U.S. states, there are no regulations that require physicians to be trained in MRI technology, nor are there regulations that require physicians to be trained in the particular body part being imaged. This means that a radiologist who works with x-ray or CT can interpret an MRI exam, and that a radiologist who specializes in neuroanatomy can read an MRI exam of the breast. It also means that any physician—even one with no training in imaging—can officially write the written report summarizing the content of a medical image in the majority of U.S. states.

Although interpretation of images by an unskilled practitioner is uncommon, it does occur. Some of the technologists I interviewed expressed concern over this practice. One technologist related a situation in which she had created an exam of a patient's pelvis and was astounded by the obvious misinterpretation of its content by a radiologist. Her concern over the quality of the written report caused her to investigate the identity of its author. She explained, "I researched who read the exam and it was a neuroradiologist. A neuroradiologist shouldn't be reading a pelvic exam. But he was the radiologist on duty that day and instead of saying that he was incompetent to read it, he read the exam." There is currently no formal regulation that limits

---

This Act was authorized in 1992 and reauthorized in 1998 by the U.S. Congress. The links between the creation of this legislation and various interest groups, such as breast cancer activist organizations, have yet to be fully investigated.

physicians from doing this. This lack of regulation, like the other policies that guide interpretation work, shapes MRI exams, and promotes varied interpretation practices.

In all, institutional practices and polices in the United States emphasize speed, revenue, and low-quality interpretations of exams. Tropes used to discuss this technology in the public sphere erase the broader political and social contexts that prioritize speed and revenue. Indeed, all of the relations and decisions that support, constrain, and inform the social construction of MRI exams are rendered invisible by hegemonic language practices that position medical images as objective and authoritative knowledge.

Social science scholarship has yet to fully investigate how routine health care policies are developed and maintained (see, e.g., Abraham and Sheppard 1999; Allen 2003; Martin and Richards 1995; Timmermans and Leiter 2000). While science and technology studies (STS) work carefully analyzes how various actors construct and mobilize definitions of science and expertise to participate in the creation of policies about controversial technoscientific practices, there is little research that addresses publicly accepted regulations.[16] As Susan Cozzens and Edward Woodhouse (1995, 552) provokingly ask, "Ought STS to devote more effort to the study of the structural mobilization of bias, that is, to the issues that do *not* become controversial?" The analysis of MRI provides one approach to the mobilization of bias and the maintenance of routine policies and practices in health care.

Linking analyses of institutional contexts, work practices, and public discourses demonstrates how common rhetorical strategies do not stay contained in popular culture or mass media. These narratives have political effects in policy and regulation as well. Tropes that equate the MRI scan with transparency, certainty, and progress do not *cause* current policies and institutional practices, but they do help sustain and reinforce them by erasing knowledge of the relationships that shape the production and use of MRI exams. This erasure contributes to the production of uncontroversial science, making it more difficult for patients, health care

---

[16] Within STS, controversial technologies and scientific claims are those that are contested by the public, scientists, or members of both groups. Uncontroversial science refers to technologies or claims that are taken for granted or accepted by many people (e.g., scientists, members of the public). In these cases, there is little public discussion about their use. By examining uncontroversial science, scholars can investigate the ideas, policies, and practices that keep such technologies or claims from being contested. Such work can transform taken for granted technologies or scientific practices into subjects for debate and discussion. For an overview of different STS approaches to policy and controversial science and technology, see Martin and Richards (1995).

professionals, and policy makers to question or intervene in current health care practices.

While other factors such as the professional authority of physicians and the pressure to contain health care costs share in the creation and maintenance of current policies, the ideas produced by popular discourses are powerful cultural forces. Through the simultaneous production of a particular view of medical images and erasure of other perspectives, popular narratives naturalize the idea that images "reveal" the inner body, making it acceptable that there are no regulations about the choices used to create an MRI exam. These narratives also support policies that suggest interpreting an image is an easy, straightforward process. Regulations in most areas of the United States presently state that any physician, indeed only one physician, is necessary to translate an exam into a written report. They do not need any particular training to do this. This practice can appear reasonable only in a symbolic milieu that aligns the image with transparency and truth.

Signifying Truth: Visuality, Technology, and the Body

As we move further into the twenty-first century, imaging will increasingly occupy both medical practice and cultural imaginations of the body. Today, images produced by high-tech machines have remarkable status and operate as signifiers of authoritative knowledge. Across social worlds, medical images are thought to represent transparency, impartiality, and truth about the human body. On close examination of discursive texts and medical practices, the symbolic positioning of these technovisual products produces an erasure of the multiple forces, decisions, and contexts that influence the content and use of medical images. This symbolic positioning further erases how what counts as truth and authoritative knowledge change across time, disciplinary boundaries, and social contexts.

Popular narratives about MRI do not draw from local knowledges and practices of the technology. Instead, these accounts reflect and reinforce popular cultural assumptions about images and machines. MRI exams, in all their complexity, are represented as accurate anatomical pictures produced through the use of technology; that is, they are embedded in ideologies that equate visual representations with the real and mechanical reproduction with objectivity. Presented as images, MRI exams are surrounded by the myth of photographic truth and rhetorical practices that suggest the picture and the real are interchangeable, instead of co-constitutive of each other.

The use of the technology itself is, of course, consequential. MRI exams, or at least the images and meanings they create, are produced through the use of technology. Machines currently occupy a privileged space in the cultural production of objectivity and truth. Human decisions are no longer compatible with notions of objectivity; the machine connotes neutrality in the production of knowledge. Culturally positioned as free of human intervention, technologies—especially expensive and complicated ones— are understood as crucial to the production of rigorous knowledge.

The visual and the technological combined thus evoke broader cultural meanings that bolster and normalize rhetorical patterns and beliefs that equate the MRI exam with transparency and objective knowledge. Indeed, discursive practices that equate the image with the real are so commonplace that even physicians and technologists use them in conversation with colleagues and others. Of course, these practitioners are acutely aware that medical images are shaped by individual decisions and institutional contexts, yet the power of normative beliefs about medical images shapes the discourse of these social actors.[17] Although local contexts may cause scientists, physicians, or consumers to reject hegemonic narratives about images and technology, the general symbolic economy forges links among mechanical reproduction, images, and transparency, which in turn shapes common discursive patterns, consumer practices, and policies.

Seeing does not equal truth or unmediated access to the human body. While cultural beliefs equate technologically produced images of the body with both the physical body itself and authoritative knowledge, these beliefs are not immune from instability or critique. Local knowledge of work practices demonstrates how MRI exams etch together aspects of the physical body, decisions by technologists and physicians, and economic and social contexts to constitute a particular and situated body in medical practice and social life.

Chapter 4 explores how the current emphasis on productivity and the professional hierarchies between physicians and technologists shape the organization and experience of work in imaging units. Studying work practices further illustrates the broader social trends and relations that produce MRI in practice.

[17] Joseph Dumit (1999) shows how cultural beliefs about mechanically produced pictures influence the discourse and actions of judges in U.S. courtrooms. While some judges control and manage the use of brain images to combat the potential effects of these views on jurors' interpretation practices, other judges are less reflective about the presence and effects of cultural beliefs that equate images with truth. These judges allow jurors to view brain scans without an explanation of the theories that connect them to medical diagnoses, reinforcing the idea that images provide transparent knowledge about the body and identity (1999, 191).

The Image Factory

Work Practices in MRI Units

Commodities. Factories. Assembly lines. We do not usually associate these words with the production of MRI exams. Examinations are instead typically described as pictures, tests, or information, and radiologists and technologists are understood as health care professionals. Such labels encourage us to think that MRI examinations exist outside of the realm of production and capital. They do not. Salaries, cost, and working conditions—although seldom discussed in the public realm—are integral to the production of the image as knowledge, and these workplace issues contribute to the social shaping of medical technologies.

Technologists and radiologists do not occupy a simple, white-collar world of information transfer; they can also be viewed as workers on an assembly line who create commodities—MRI examinations—for mass consumption. Invoking the word *commodities* relocates anatomical images in a system of exchange—one that is populated by human beings and increasingly subject to the mass production techniques of repetition and mechanization. These techniques are used to generate volume, but human beings provide the material from which the commodities—MRI scans—are made. The emphasis on process and volume informs production in all parts of American life, and the creation of medical knowledge takes place in this broader context.

Theorizing the imaging unit as labor provokes the following questions: How do contemporary notions of efficiency shape the organization of work and care in MRI units? How do technologists and radiologists understand—and can they resist—the increasing mechanization of their work? How are the social and economic hierarchies between physicians and technologists related to the experience of work and the implementation of assembly-line techniques? And, how is safety, which is a key issue for workers, defined and experienced by technologists and radiologists? This chapter illustrates how technologists and radiologists creatively negotiate patient care, work hierarchies, and issues of safety even while subject to the increasing mechanization of medical knowledge production.

Enter the Image Assembly Line

Using a complex array of computer equipment, magnets, and coils that is collectively known as MRI technology, technologists and radiologists produce MRI examinations. They create and interpret images through repetitive, mechanized processes on the medical knowledge assembly line. In the first stage of production, technologists repeat specialized tasks and work quickly to translate the physical body into a series of pictorial objects. Once this is accomplished, radiologists or other physicians then perform the work of interpreting these images.

Technologists are highly skilled individuals who work closely with technoscientific knowledge and apparatuses. Still, the training of technologists is not federally regulated, and most states do not require MRI technologists to be licensed. Most employers do require technologists to complete a two-year radiologic technologist (RT) program, and some expect technologists to also pass the MRI specialization examination offered by the American Registry of Radiologic Technologists (ARRT).[1]

MRI exams begin when technologists, usually dressed in scrubs or regular clothes covered by a white hospital coat, meet with patients who are usually dressed in hospital gowns. During this initial encounter, technologists interview patients to ensure their safety during the examination. Screening questions such as "Metal in the body?" and "Do you have a pacemaker?" are asked. The magnetic field produced by an MRI system will pull metal objects—even those located in a person's body—toward the

---

[1] By 2006, 16,698 registered technologists (RTs) had passed the MRI registry exam, but as many as 32,000 individuals may actually work in MRI units (American Registry of Radiologic Technologists [ARRT] 2006; Harris 2006). Most technologists, including those who complete an RT program, get their primary training on the job where they learn the trade through practice and interaction with colleagues. However, the professionalization of technologists is beginning to occur. Development of programs that specifically train people in MRI technology are in process. It is too soon to know how or if formal educational requirements will be developed for MRI technologists.

machine, causing harm to the individual. It can also alter the pacing of pacemakers, leading them to malfunction. During the exchange, technologists may also give an overview of the exam, answer questions, and address concerns voiced by patients. Lack of time often prevents this discussion from going into detail.

After completing the screening procedure, patients get onto a stretcherlike platform, and the technologists press the button that slides patients into the MRI machine. The technologists then leave the room and sit at a computer desk in an adjacent room. The computer area where technologists work is generally dark so that they can better see the screen. There is also a small window so that they can watch the person in the machine. The temperature in the room is kept cool for the maintenance of electronic equipment such as computers.

During an exam, technologists talk to patients via a microphone between scans. "How are you doing? The next scan is six minutes. Hold still." An examination can last anywhere from twenty minutes to an hour and includes multiple scans of the body part under investigation. After the scans are obtained, the technologists escort patients back to the dressing room, and either print out the resulting images on film for the radiologists or send them to the radiologists in electronic format via computer networks.

Like other assembly-line occupations, the technologist's job is based on *repetition* and *specialization*—two techniques that promote the flow of patients through the imaging unit. Technologists replicate the entire sequence of actions from screening to printing throughout the day and (at some locations) night, as they work on and with machines to transform parts of patients' bodies into a series of images. These images become the body—or at least one of the bodies—encountered by the referring physician who then sorts through different test results to formulate a diagnosis and treatment plan (Mol 2002).

The use of factory techniques permeates the work experiences of technologists. The speed, or what some might call the "efficiency," of factory production comes from breaking down processes into repetitive tasks that focus a worker's attention on a component of the whole. The fragmentation of production practices complements the fragmentation of the body in the examination; each mutually reinforces the other to create an assembly-line perspective that emphasizes the part and the task, not the whole. The technologists themselves have adopted language that emphasizes the fragmentary nature of their work. In my fieldwork, I observed how technologists referred to patients as body parts. Statements like, "I have a liver sitting outside," "I just put a brain on the table," and "Is the breast here yet?" were commonly used to discuss people waiting for MRI examinations.

The centrality of mass production techniques is also evident in the use of other factory-related language such as "throughput," "move-ups," and "add-ons." In factory work, *throughput* refers to the amount of raw material processed by an industrial plant in a given amount of time. More recently, it is used in computer industries to refer to the amount of data processed by a computer over a stated time period. In imaging units, *throughput* refers to the movement of patients through the scanner. *Move-ups*, a phrase created by health care workers to reflect the flexible, human assembly line, refers to patients who are rescheduled for earlier appointments. *Add-ons*, another innovative term, describes people who need an examination but are not yet scheduled. This terminology signals the value placed on work flow and reflects the transformation of humans into objects that may be more easily processed.

Acceleration of Production

Speed, a crucial element of factory labor, is another important component to the structure of work in an MRI facility. Automobile manufacturer Henry Ford, one of the first to apply assembly-line techniques to mass production, increased the speed of production as a way to produce more and more yield. In his biography of Ford, Keith Sward (1948) admiringly discusses the assembly line and Ford's use of "speed-ups": "By 1930, therefore, the only way to run this remarkable and almost perfect apparatus [the assembly line] cheaper was to run it faster, just as it stood. On the line this meant additional pure man speed-up, or in the language of the shop, lowering costs by 'taking it out of the men'" (354). Taking it out of the "men" means that it is workers—both men and women—who bear the brunt of this strategy. However, the use of speed-ups in health care affects more than workers. Patients, the raw material on the assembly line, suffer the consequences of emphasizing speed over quality of care.

The technologists at the sites I observed were similarly pressured to increase the volume of patients scanned. As one technologist explained, "I think that hospitals and a lot of places are interested in turnover. Get them in. Get them out. Get them in. Get them out. Get them in. Get them out." Another technologist said, "Techs are under more pressure now to do faster exams. Since scans are quicker, techs are expected to do exams in thirty minutes instead of sixty minutes." As another technologist noted, "There is so much work going on these days, we're going so fast and putting people in and out, in and out." Moving bodies in and out as quickly as possible is the goal.

As part of the process of acceleration, technologists in hospital settings are expected to fill any cancellations.[2] If free time opens up at hospital MRI units, technologists are supposed to locate another potential patient. They search waiting lists or call other wards in the hospital to find someone to fill the vacant spot. The taboo against the machine standing empty is directly enforced through conversations among technologists, physicians, and managers and indirectly enforced by the sense that a supervisor or physician could walk by at anytime. The command to fill vacancies creates a certain amount of chaos. In my fieldword, voices often called out, "Do you have any openings?" and phones rang constantly as receptionists called to see if any space had opened up.

Technologists have to move bodies—both their own and patients—faster. The subjective experience of the emphasis on speed and volume is one of stress and anxiety. One technologist articulated this when she said, "It is stressful doing more patients . . . you are required to do more in a shorter period of time." The pressure to speed up the movement of patients through the assembly line is compounded by the demands of working with ill individuals, who often move slowly if they are injured or do not feel well. Patients are often taken aback when they realize they have to lie inside the machine. As one technologist explained, "It is hard. The administration doesn't realize the test might take 20 minutes but it might take you 10 minutes just to talk them [patients] into going into the magnet. They don't want to look at issues like that." Or, as another technologist noted, "This [faster exams] is not realistic. It can take time getting an in-patient or uncomfortable patient into the scanner." A tension exists between the pressure technologists feel to process more patients and the emotional support technologists have to and want to give to patients.

While individual institutions may put colorful pictures or fake plants in the examination room to create a soothing environment, these additions often stand in stark juxtaposition to the value placed on repetition and speed. In one of the places I observed, an artificial *Ficus* plant stood askew in a corner of the examination room. It had been pushed aside to make room for an emergency, and it was not returned to its original location during my weeks of fieldwork.

The demand to speed up the process permeates technologists' consciousness. One technologist eloquently illustrated how acceleration has become a way to understand change and work when he discussed the

[2] Technologists at freestanding clinics are not under the same constraints as technologists at hospital units because large quantities of immediately accessible patients do not exist in free standing facilities.

recent shift in MRI terminology. Over the past few years, people in the medical and manufacturing/sales communities have shortened the name MRI to MR and the technology is often called MR in these circles. Explaining the linguistic change through an understanding of the acceleration of production, the technologist noted, correctly or not, "I think it is MR because it is less words. We have got to move faster."[3]

Designing the "Efficient" Imaging Unit

The way in which MRI units are designed also affects the speed with which patients flow through a facility. MRI units are often designed so that the computer screen faces away from the path patients take as they exit the examination room. This design prevents patients from stopping to view images as they leave, a curiosity that slows down work flow. As one technologist explained, "We are on a really tight schedule. You just don't have that type of time [to show patients the images]. I know it sounds kind of cold, but we really don't have time."

Another less common design used to facilitate flow is the addition of a door that allows patients to bypass the computer area. In this layout, two doors go into the examination room. One door, used by the technologist, connects the examination room to the room with the computer. The other door, for the patient, leads from the dressing room directly into the exam room. With this design, the patient never enters the control room, which prevents patients from seeing and thus asking about their scans. One technologist who worked in an MRI unit that used the two-door design said, "Patients never asked, never were concerned [with their images]. They never had the inkling to look over." For the sake of efficiency, production takes precedence over patients' desire to see and learn about their own health and anatomy.

Docile Patients

Humans, like the raw materials on the Ford assembly line, can and do disrupt production on the imaging assembly line. Whether they react with anxiety or curiosity, people can slow down the process of getting an MRI.

---

[3] Marketing reasons contribute to the shortening of the name (e.g., changing MRI to MR). The new terminology opens up the possibility of marketing specialized equipment such as magnetic resonance angiography (MRA) or magnetic resonance spectroscopy (MRS).

Accelerating the process means making patients more cooperative, or, as philosopher Michel Foucault (1979) suggests, producing "docile bodies." Docile bodies are disciplined and follow the strict routines of daily life. Producing docile patients takes work because people are anything but docile in their initial encounters with MRI technology. The nature of MRI procedures—their length, loudness, and the positioning of the body inside the machine—causes patients to resist docility.

Not surprisingly, people often react strongly to the machine. The potential danger of the technology requires bold warning signs to be placed around the entrance to the MRI room and patients to undergo strict screening procedures before entering this area. In addition to this heightened awareness of risk, patients are placed inside the machine and are expected to lie still in this chamber for the duration of the examination. Since exams can last anywhere from twenty to sixty minutes, people are enclosed in a physical state of stillness for an extended period of time. The stillness and sense of enclosure are further compounded by the loud knocking sound produced when the machine is in use. Reminiscent of a train passing by, a rumbling noise reverberates throughout the room while the exam is in process. The mix of sensory deprivation and sensory overload makes the experience of having an exam unsettling and memorable.

Referring physicians, radiologists, and technologists alike acknowledge how powerfully the experience affects them. One physician captured the intensity of an examination when he described his own experience as a patient: "You are really enclosed. It's noisy. Buzzings and things. Growling. It [the exam] took about forty-five minutes, and you are laying there with this thing right in front of your face. You're pretty much sensory deprived except for this noise. . . [pauses] I was laying there thinking that if I were the least bit claustrophobic or the least bit demented I can see how this would tip you over the edge." Another radiologist highlighted what he called the dehumanizing effect of the examination: "I felt disoriented. After about fifteen minutes I couldn't tell which was up or down or right or left, I sort of feel disoriented. I had a head coil on, which is also, I think, very dehumanizing. It looks like a hockey mask, and you're in a tube." The combination of the enclosure in the machine with a coil on his face took away this physician's sense of humanity and transformed him into a part of the technology itself.

Even technologists who work closely with the machine talk about the extreme experience of an exam. One technologist recalled her first exam—one that she had before she became a technologist: "You don't know how the technology works, you don't have the background, you don't know what's going on, there's this big huge—you're in this tunnel, you're alone in the room, it's making a lot of noise. It's frightening, it really is."

Although many people find ways to manage the sensory discomfort that accompanies an MRI examination, others do not. The feeling of enclosure, the loud noise, the sensory deprivation—all these factors make it hard for some people to complete the exam. Exam incompletion is a well-recognized problem in the MRI community. Numerous studies evaluate the reasons why patients are unable to complete an MRI (primarily anxiety and claustrophobia) and recommend strategies to deal with them (Melendez and McCrank 1993; Skler et al. 1991; Thorpe et al. 1990). One psychologist, Paul Friday, even created the name "failed scan syndrome" (FSS) to describe uncompleted examinations (Segal 1995).

Technologists, physicians, and machine designers creatively and intensively work to transform patients into compliant bodies. In the early and mid-1990s, technologists primarily used relaxation strategies such as talking to patients during the exam, offering patients headphones to listen to music, and providing aromatherapy to soothe anxiety and facilitate patient flow. Such strategies may or may not produce the docility needed to complete the examination. Medication is another intervention now used: people who are claustrophobic or extremely anxious may be mildly sedated prior to an examination. While methods such as headphones and talk are still used for routine situations, sedatives are more quickly administered if patients think they will have a problem. Drug-induced sedation secures a completed examination, which benefits both patients, who get information from the test, and the imaging unit, which keeps the patient-object in motion and allows productivity to increase. This strategy shifts the time burden from the technologist to the patient, who now has to come in earlier for the sedation and stay later to recover from it.

The open MRI machine also facilitates compliance and enhances productivity. In 1989, Hitachi pioneered the open MRI machine, and by the mid-1990s other imaging manufacturers produced this design as well. The machine, as its name suggests, has open side walls. The person being scanned still lies sandwiched in the middle of the machine, but two of the surrounding walls are now open. Open machines initially used a weaker magnet than the one used in the standard or closed MRI machines. Since magnet strength is related to image quality, open MRI machines were criticized for producing lower-quality images. In 2005, manufacturers released open MRI machines that use a high-field magnet similar to the type used in closed machines. The new machines address the quality concerns raised about previous open machines and may mean that patients can have an open MRI examination without compromising resolution quality.

Other design innovations such as lower table heights and providing more room between the patient and the machine walls in closed machines make people more comfortable during the exam. Such technological solutions aim to alleviate anxious reactions to the MRI technology and ensure exam completion.

Defining a "Good" Exam Experience

Music, talk, sedation, and technology design are all possible strategies to soothe anxiety and facilitate patient flow. No one method ensures patient compliance and exam completion. However, the values embedded in definitions of what makes a good examination are worth considering. A technologist I interviewed offered insight into what makes a good examination experience: "There was an article in an x-ray magazine about a patient who had the same test two weeks apart. The first technologist was wonderful and explained everything and let somebody in the room with them and this and that. The next time he had another technologist, same type of exam. No. They can't come in the room with you. Just didn't explain. And from a patient's point of view the difference was terrible. The experience he had the second time was terrible, and it just was little things a technologist could have done."

Drawing on the article and her own work experience, the technologist outlined three things that make patients more comfortable and help them complete the exam. First, patients feel more secure when a friend or family member is in the room with them. "I think it's better if they [patients] have somebody in the room with them. They'd feel a lot better when there's another person right there," she explained. Second, patients feel reassured when technologists talk with them and offer some forms of professional body contact such as touching the head. "If you talk to them a lot. Give them a lot of body contact. Even if their head is out, touch their head," she recommended. Finally, technologists need to demonstrate empathy, letting patients know that they understand how they might be feeling. This technologist recommended acknowledging the stress of an exam to build a connection with patients.

While the new open MRI machines and other design innovations hold promise for creating a more manageable patient experience, it will take hospitals and freestanding imaging centers time to change over to the new machines. In the meantime, technologists can make exams more comfortable for patients through talk, touch, and empathy, all of which are forms of emotional labor that are devalued in an operation that assigns high value to work flow and volume.

Into the Reading Room

The reading room is the name given to the room where the radiologists interpret or read MRI examinations, verbally transforming image content into pathology and normal anatomy. Transcribers, located in yet another site, translate and at times edit the radiologist's verbal recording into a written report, which is then sent to the referring physician.

As with technologists, there are no laws requiring radiologists to have any formal education or certification in MRI technology. In fact, as noted in chapter 3, any MD or DO, with training or not, can legally interpret MRI examinations with or without training.

Of all workers on the assembly line, radiologists are the most invisible to patients, and, unless the referring doctors stress it, their contributions to the production process can go unnoticed. Patients seldom meet radiologists, who come into the exam room only if there is a problem or a procedure that requires assistance. The typical patient interacts only with the technologist during the exam.

Like technologists, radiologists function in an assembly-line format, and their work is repetitive. In larger hospitals, they sit side by side in the reading room, quietly murmuring their interpretations into the red record light on the microphone. In smaller centers, they primarily work alone. While they may call in the technologists on site or phone another physician if stumped or impressed by an unusual scan, radiologists at freestanding centers or small hospitals typically transform images into verbal recordings on their own. The pictures are the central focus of this part of the assembly line, and the reading room is usually dimly lit so that physicians can concentrate on them.

Specialization is another key component of their assembly-line work. Although radiologists who work in rural or small hospitals may interpret the output of many visualization technologies and focus on a wide range of anatomy, there is a broader trend toward fragmentation and specialization. In freestanding imaging centers and large hospitals, radiologists typically interpret a range of anatomy, but will focus on the output of one technology (e.g., ultrasound, CT, MRI). At larger imaging sites, the work of radiologists can be even more specialized. In these cases, radiologists may concentrate on one particular imaging technique and/or on one area of the body. Radiologists who want to work in a university hospital environment and interpret the output of various visualization technologies and a range of anatomy often have difficulty finding positions that offer this flexibility.

Along with repetition and fragmentation, work in radiology is often marked by an increase in volume in terms of both the number and complexity of examinations. Each MRI exam includes a series of pictures. While both routine and complex exams include multiple images, complex exams can produce even more images, and they can also involve additional techniques such as the use of a contrast medium. At one site I observed, radiologists read between twenty and forty-five exams per day, a figure that is up from previous years. Of these exams, many were also more complex and required more work by the radiologist. The trend of increasing average workload per radiologist is taking place across many sites in the United States (Lu and Arenson 2006; Matin et al. 2006). One study showed, for example, that "for nearly every analyzed category and subcategory of radiologists, there was an increase in average annual number of procedures per FTE [full-time equivalent] radiologist" since 1991 (Bhargavan and Sunshine 2005, 926). Radiologists who work with MRI in particular experience significant increases in workload, which is due in part to rapid growth in the technology's use (Applegate and Rumack 2003).

The radiologists I interviewed are well aware of the transformation in productivity, and some talked about it openly. For example, when I asked one radiologist if there was pressure from the hospital administration to see patients quickly, he responded, "Yeah. Well, to see lots of patients. Doesn't matter how long you take. It's the volume they want." Radiologists can choose how long to spend with a particular case or to stay longer at work if they want to spend more time on examinations. What counts is overall volume. As another radiologist stated, "Over the past few years productivity has become more of an issue."

Other radiologists discussed the reasons for increased volume. For example, one radiologist attributed it to the time pressures experienced by referring doctors as they too are expected to see more patients. He explained, "I think MR has become a screening modality. I think it used to be, when it first came out, was sort of like something that if you have a question on other modalities, you want to further evaluate it, then you do MRI. But, now, I think because the pressure of time on the referrals [referring doctors], because 'why should I do a long physical exam when I can just image and see what is there?'" He added that the increase in volume of MRI scans occurs "Because the population is aging; there are more people who are sick, more chronic disease. You have less and less time. And not accounting for the hospitals or whatever, trying to shorten the amount of time you have to see more patients." For another radiologist, MRI use is increasing "because it makes money." The fee-for-service reimbursement system ensures that each procedure ordered or patient seen generates revenue, which creates an incentive to use procedures and see more patients.

The increase in volume affects radiologists and technologists differently. Radiologists have more control over the way they accomplish their work. Radiologists have a list of examinations that need to be interpreted that day. Within that constraint, they can choose when and how long to spend on each case as well as the order of exam interpretation. They can also choose when and why to take breaks. Radiologists' work is independent of patient flow. Patients in the waiting room do not get backlogged if there is a delay in interpretation.

Radiologists also have more control over their schedule because they primarily work for themselves as individuals or in groups distinct from the hospital or imaging center, and they can decide how much they want to earn. This occurs because radiologists receive income from health insurance providers or from patients for each procedure performed. Those who work by themselves receive the money generated by reading fees, the professional component of imaging bills. For those in radiology groups, salaries come from the pooled income obtained by these fees, which are then distributed to members of that group.

Radiologists can thus partly control production pressures by deciding to hire more physicians, but that would mean less income for each radiologist. One doctor explained how radiology groups negotiate productivity:

> How much pressure we are under is partly a function of our own group. We are not hospital employees. We are an independent group. So how much stress we are under is partly a function of how big we want to be. A large component of our practice is fee for service. So if you want to read more, you get more. If you read less, you get less. And so we have a fairly compatible group in terms of how hard we want to work and some groups work harder and some groups don't work as hard.

Thus, the group decides what is acceptable volume (and thus income), and members comply.

While radiologists have control over the increase in production and the financial benefit that comes from increased volume, technologists are wage laborers who cannot decide on their own how to divide the labor among more workers. Such decisions are made by hospital administrators or unit managers who may or may not consult technologists. As wage laborers for hospitals and imaging centers, technologists have wages that stay the same regardless of the number of examinations completed. Any income generated from the increased productivity of technologists is used to offset other hospital costs or to supplement the income of the owners of private imaging centers.

Radiologists, however, do not have complete control over production. Diminishing reimbursement rates, a common trend in medicine, require radiologists to increase volume to maintain their standard of living. Reimbursement fees are typically at their highest when a medical technique is first introduced to clinical practice. This occurs because physicians and administrators primarily set the fee and there is little competition from other suppliers. As time passes, health insurance providers, especially through the efforts of Medicaid and Medicare representatives, decrease what they are willing to pay for a particular procedure. This change, coupled with the increasing availability of a procedure, bring down reimbursement rates, which means physicians must perform more procedures to maintain the same income. "We do ultimately feel it because there is a tendency to squeeze and if you want to maintain a certain income level, you certainly have to be more productive than in the past," a radiologist explained. Here, a tendency to squeeze refers to lower reimbursement rates.

In addition to approaching their work with an emphasis on production and efficiency, radiologists have also adopted assembly-line language to describe what they do. Like technologists, the radiologists I interviewed discussed their work in terms of productivity, volume, and efficiency. During one conversation, for example, a radiologist used factory metaphors to discuss trade-offs between using an open machine, which can potentially decrease the length of an exam since less time is spent soothing patients' anxiety, and the fact that open machines usually have low-field magnets. Lower-field magnets require that patients spend more time in the machine to get an acceptable image. "You know ironically, you think open magnets, it's not really a shortcut, because the exam takes longer because the magnet is lower field strength," he said. "So it's not a throughput thing. It's not like the radiologist can say, 'Oh I have an open magnet. I can bang people through.'" Even though open MRI machines may require less patient management, radiologists are unable to "bang people through."

Radiologists frequently discussed ways to decrease the length of exams as a way to increase efficiency and productivity. One radiologist noted,

"I have tried to cut back here. Become more cost-effective. I came from a practice where we did three patients per hour on the magnet. Here we do one every forty-five minutes." Other radiologists also thought in terms of money and productivity; one explained, "Every day the magnet didn't generate income, we're losing money." Use of economic terminology signals that physicians are aware of the emphasis on production and think about their work in these terms.

Another group also benefits from shorter examinations: patients. Yet while patients certainly prefer a shorter stay at an MRI facility and in an MRI machine, their experience was seldom mentioned as a reason to cut the length of an exam. Only one physician mentioned that shorter exams are more comfortable for patients. The majority of physicians I interviewed evaluated the length of the scan through the lens of cost and efficiency.

The Negotiation and Resistance of Production Processes

Despite the broader institutional emphasis on production, technologists and radiologists resist reducing their work to a question of volume, speed, and repetition. Technologists, for example, interact with patients on an emotional level despite the emphasis on speed and productivity. In fact, the technologists I interviewed and observed considered emotional labor an essential part of the job. As one technologist explained, "Definitely number one in radiology, in anything, it should be compassion. That's a big plus for patients when they come in. They are scared. I think that needs to be number one." Working with patients who have been or are about to be diagnosed with cancer or other serious illnesses requires strong interpersonal skills. The technologists I interviewed valued this aspect of their job even though work conditions made it harder to implement.

The emotional labor of technologists also challenged assumptions about masculinity. Men constitute approximately 40 percent of MRI technologists, which contrasts with other imaging fields such as x-ray or ultrasound where they represent approximately 25 percent (Harris 2006). In addition, the work of technologists includes lifting bodies, understanding science, and commanding complicated technology—all activities broadly perceived as masculine. Thus, MRI technologists engage in activities understood as masculine yet value and perform caregiving work. This active emotional labor occurs despite cultural understandings that link bodies and activities coded as masculine to intellectual or physical rather than emotional work.

The importance of emotional labor is recognized in the training programs for technologists and degree requirements. In the radiologic technologist (RT) degree program, students take courses that develop caregiving skills. Such courses teach technologists to understand the diversity of patients' experiences and provide strategies to enhance patient comfort. Explaining his training, one technologist noted, "They [the teachers] give you scenarios about patients. Say a patient has to fast 24 hours for a test. Then don't walk through with food. Little things like that that you might not think of." Program literature also emphasizes "competent, concerned patient care" (see, e.g., Department of Radiation Sciences [DRS] 2006), and professional associations highlight "relationship centered patient care" as well as other components of the job such as the development of scientific and technical skills (ASRT 2006, 4).

In my fieldwork, technologists demonstrated a strong commitment to doing emotional work. This commitment could be seen in the way technologists interacted with patients. Between scans, for example, they would ask the patients how they were doing and offer words of encouragement. A typical phrase was "The next scan will be four minutes. You are doing great." After an exam was completed, technologists took the time to let the patient reorient themselves before helping them on their way. They often used professional forms of touch to help people balance and feel connected. Other evidence of the workers' commitment to emotional care was seen in their consideration of patients' emotional needs. One member of the staff, for instance, brought plastic rosary beads into work so that Catholic patients could bring them into the magnet if they desired. This person explained to me that he thought of doing this after a nun had come in for an examination. The nun brought her rosary beads to help her through the exam, but they contained metal so she was unable to bring them into the machine. The nun's experience caused the worker to wonder how the emotional needs of Catholic patients could be taken into account should the situation arise again. On his own time, he bought plastic rosary beads and brought them to work. The technologist's sympathy for and willingness to use his own time to address the emotional needs of patients was mirrored by other technologists who took care of patients' well-being in a myriad of ways. The ability of most technologists to do emotional labor in a system that primarily recognizes speed and volume is notable.

In the text *Making Gray Gold: Narratives of Nursing Home Care*, sociologist Timothy Diamond (1992) discusses the erasure of emotional work in health care, focusing on the work practices of aides in nursing homes. He notes that the belief "If it's not charted, it didn't happen," structures work in these sites (131). According to Diamond (166), the emphasis on the chart "erased work such as waiting for someone to make an endlessly slow walk down the hall or knowing how to touch someone in the right spots and not to touch someone else in the wrong ones . . . No terms connected with caring, relations, or emotions found their way here to muddy up the smooth, carefully calculated records of care. The job was organizationally produced as menial and mechanical, industrially streamlined to complement the making of patients."

The tendency to erase emotional work supports the decision to run nursing homes based on schedules and routine. The needs of the humans involved, whether workers or clients, are not taken into account. Like the technologists at the MRI centers I observed, the aides at the nursing homes Diamond observed try to practice emotional work. Both groups, however, have to fit this in around the demands of the productive work schedule—demands which do not take this type of labor into account, never mind reward it.

In addition to challenging the devaluation of emotional labor, technologists also resisted the way in which the organization of their labor reduced them to a cog in the machine. Wherever there was room for creativity, technologists often took advantage of it. Technologists, for example, speak to patients in the machine through a microphone on the computer keyboard. Much like radio deejays, technologists develop their own personal style to communicate with the patients via the audio technology. One technologist, for example, used a soothing, deep voice to speak to the individuals in the machine. Another used a booming, welcome-to-the-carnival type of voice. This man would lengthen vowels stretching the words out. "Alrighty," he'd say. "Take a deep breath. Take another deep breath, and hold it." These voices were not used when interacting with patients face to face. Instead, they were personas created by the technologists, sometimes consciously, sometimes unconsciously, in a particular situation.

The radiologists I encountered also resisted the mechanization of their labor. For them, however, the primary way of resisting was not engaging in emotional labor with patients given that radiologists seldom encounter actual patients. Instead, radiologists tried to avoid repetition and fragmentation when tending to their professional tasks.

I interviewed radiologists who worked at private imaging centers and small hospitals, as well as those who worked at large university-affiliated hospitals. The radiologists employed at university-affiliated hospitals challenged the monotony of repetitive work by taking jobs at academic institutions instead of working in other types of settings. Such positions allowed them to expand their labor to include research and teaching as well as image interpretation. University-based radiologists take a significant cut in pay in exchange for being able to do varied tasks, but the ones I spoke with felt that, for the most part, it was well worth it. They got to conduct research on new imaging applications and think about medical imaging from the perspectives of residents, referring physicians, and policy makers. Medical workers and policy makers all count on the work done by university radiologists as their research furthers the field and evaluates changes in imaging use.

Other radiologists countered the emphasis on volume by choosing group practices that agree to accept a patient load that allows them to work at a reasonable pace. As noted earlier, radiology groups can set the pace of their work by deciding how many physicians will share the total income generated. Some groups choose to earn less by hiring more physicians. By doing this, such groups choose to value the pace of work over increases in income.

Radiologists from all types of employment structures bring individuality and creativity into their written reports in an effort to defy the mechanization of work. Although the general format of the report is standardized, the radiologists' choice of words and overall interpretation allow individual expression. One radiologist, for example, went for dramatic and unusual interpretations. When he interpreted an image, he looked for something that would make his report stand out. He might point out an unusual anatomical finding that does not affect the individual's health. Another radiologist individualized his reports by pointing out "a little something extra" and used colorful language to do so. Summing up the desire to add uniqueness to the otherwise monotonous task of writing reports, a radiologist explained, "Each radiologist has their own style. You can usually pick out who did a report."

Technologists and radiologists find multiple ways to resist the mechanization of their work. For these groups, there is not one form of resistance, but rather a multiplicity of forms that arise from the organization of each field. In *The History of Sexuality: An Introduction,* Foucault (1990, 95–96) analyzes contemporary forms of resistance:

> There is no single locus of great Refusal, no soul of revolt, source of all rebellions, or pure law of the revolutionary. Instead there is a plurality of resistances, each of them a special case: resistances that are possible, necessary, improbable; others that are spontaneous, savage, solitary, concerted, rampant, or violent; still others that are quick to compromise, interested, or sacrificial; by definition, they can only exist in the strategic field of power relations.

For Foucault, contemporary life is marked by micro resistances that are produced by particular social relations and structures. They can be, although they often are not, united into organized revolts. "Are there no great ruptures, massive binary divisions, then?" he asks. "Occasionally, yes. But more often one is dealing with mobile and transitory points of resistance, producing cleavages in a society that shift about, fracturing unities and effecting regroupings, furrowing across individuals themselves, cutting them up and remolding them, marking off irreducible regions in them, in their bodies and minds" (1990, 95–96). Moments of resistance, which are historically and socially produced, can create cleavages that rearrange social and political alignments. Moreover, they create one's body and self in that instance.

Acts of resistance by radiologists and technologists, and the selves they construct through such actions, can be understood as responses to the institutional and professional relations in which they labor. These responses, while produced by particular social networks, also demonstrate the creativity of human actors. People choose, whether consciously or unconsciously, to engage in actions of resistance over actions of acceptance. They also choose which of the potential forms of resistance to take up. In doing so, they exercise *creativity* and *agency*—two features of disciplinary life Foucault allows for but does not emphasize. But, as Foucault rightly predicts, a united revolt has not yet occurred. Professional and economic hierarchies are two factors that prevent technologists and radiologists from joining forces to challenge the assembly-line practices that structure their work.

Professional Hierarchies: Life on the Assembly Line

As previous studies of labor have demonstrated, social hierarchies based on gender, race, age, and class structure interaction between workers (see, e.g., Blewett 1988; Garrity-Blake 1994). There are, however, differing degrees to which this occurs within and between radiologists and technologists.[4] My

[4] Sociologist Stephen Barley (1986, 1990a) examines how the introduction of CT scanners affects professional hierarchies between technologists and radiologists. Drawing on observations of two radiology departments, Barley shows that new imaging devices challenged radiologists' professional dominance because some radiologists, as CT novices, had to learn how to work with the technology. Even in these situations, though, technologists deferred to radiologists by posing questions instead of making assertions, and radiologists asserted themselves by confirming that the technologists' actions were correct. Barley also highlights hierarchies among technologists, demonstrating that CT technologists and sonographers have more autonomy than x-ray technologists.

observations suggest that although race, gender, and age shape interaction within each group, it is the professional differences (and the resulting social class differences) between the technologists and radiologists that are most salient in MRI units.[5] These professional differences are marked by a clear hierarchy, social and physical distances, and at times antagonism.

The appearance of doctor–technologist relations initially seemed egalitarian at the institutions that I observed, and radiologists and technologists often addressed each other by first names. Despite this appearance of equality, a professional, class-based hierarchy still divides radiologists and technologists. As one technologist explained, "The hierarchy is still there. Definitely. You better believe it. It's externally friendlier. But when push comes to shove, if it's the doctor's word against the tech's word, the doctor wins." The fact that the physician's view outweighs that of the technologist can also be seen in expressions of anger and irritation.

Both radiologists and technologists find imaging clinics a challenging place to work. While the emphasis is on production and volume, the unpredictability of emergencies, bodies, and complex technology often cause production to go awry. I asked two technologists how they would describe their job, and both spontaneously shouted, "Frustrating!" Granted, all workers experience frustration. But the pecking order of a unit dictates who can lose their temper when things do not go according to plan. Radiologists and referring physicians are permitted to get angry and lose their tempers in public. Furthermore, their rank in the hierarchy means that they can yell at technologists. In contrast, technologists

[5] As documented by social scientists, health care professionals and patients often rely on social categories and hierarchies to make sense of and even treat each other (see, e.g., Cruikshank 2002; Guillemin and Holmstrom 1999; Todd 1989). In such cases, health care professionals may vary interpersonal treatment of patients according to their perceived race, class, gender, ethnicity, age, or sexuality. During the months I conducted my fieldwork, I saw only two instances in which technologists talked about patients in ways that drew on and reinforced social hierarchies. One example drew on biases against larger people, and another blamed a homeless man for his economic condition. In these cases, the technologists did not alter their treatment of patients even though they expressed disparaging comments about these individuals.

The lack of overt discrimination results from multiple factors. The technologists, physicians, and secretaries at the sites I observed represented diverse age, class, sexual, ethnic, and gender identities. In addition, the technologists labored and lived in diverse settings and were surrounded by broader cultural and professional milieus that prohibit public displays of fear of difference. Finally, the workers and managers at the facilities I observed prided themselves on excellent work, which they defined as the production of high-quality MRI exams and the treatment of *all* patients in an equal and professional manner. While my presence may have played a role in the technologists' behavior, these other factors created a climate that made overt patient discrimination unacceptable.

are not allowed to shout at physicians or in public, and if they do, they risk their job.[6]

I observed this inequality repeatedly in my fieldwork. In one instance, a physician berated a technologist for finishing an examination instead of leaving it to go find a film for her. In another situation, a radiologist came into the exam room shouting, "Why isn't anybody answering the phone?! I have been trying to call this unit." The technologists who were in charge of the phone were unable to answer it because they were working with an exceptionally challenging case. Even though the radiologist saw the chaos unfolding in front of him, he continued to yell at the technologists while they tried to complete the exam. In my fieldwork, I never saw technologists lose their temper at a physician. The hierarchy of the hospital permits physicians to shout at technologists but not vice versa.

Hierarchy and Safety

Part of the job as technologist is to serve as the "safety" gatekeeper to the examination room. Gatekeepers are required because the superconducting magnet in the MRI machine causes any metal object brought into the examination room to fly swiftly toward the machine at speeds up to 40 miles an hour and stick to it. Traveling at this speed, metal objects can hurt individuals in the room, as well as damage the machine itself. If a person carrying metal objects goes into the room, the technologist is held responsible and could be fired.

Technologists are well aware of the power of the superconducting magnet, as well as their responsibility to guard it. As one technologist joked, "We are guardians of the magnet. You must respect the magnet." The technologist's use of the term *magnet* is significant. Calling attention to its most powerful component, technologists and radiologists often refer to the machine (and at times by extension the examination room) as "the magnet" and the other components and devices of the machine are forgotten. Transformed into a superhero-like entity, the magnet is a force that requires monitoring.

Interactions between technologists and other health care professionals over safety issues reflect a twist in the hierarchical structure of the medical

[6] At one site, the manager of the MRI unit explicitly supported the autonomy and authority of technologists. If a fellow or resident expressed uncalled-for anger at the technologists at this site, the manager would back the technologists' right to confront these individuals. The manager's support of the technologists helped improve the unequal power dynamic between the two groups. Nonetheless, it remains unclear whether this same manager would be able to back the technologists' viewpoints against an attending physician, or a full-time, permanent physician. Attending physicians are at the apex of hospital hierarchies, whereas residents and fellows occupy a midlevel position of expert-in-training.

workplace. As gatekeepers, technologists constantly confront physicians and nurses to ensure that they do not enter the room with metal objects. This dynamic means that technologists repeatedly challenge individuals who have more status than they do. But, due to their lower status, they are often unable to perform their job as "guardian."

One technologist recalled an incident in which a nurse ignored the technologist's safety questions:

> I remember one time a nurse came down with a critical care patient. She was very quick with me. Very irritated. I know I had asked her about scissors and everything, because they [the nurses] are always carrying scissors around. She went around to the back of the magnet. The patient was in the magnet and I heard this "clang." I'm like, "What was that?" "Oh, just my scissors." And I am like "Thank God it didn't hit the patient." But it stuck to the side and I was able to grab it off. I just wanted to shake her. She could have hurt the patient. I am watching out for all of our welfare.

The technologist's lower status in the interaction meant that (1) the technologist had to negotiate the nurse's irritability while simultaneously trying to screen the nurse for entrance into the unit and (2) the nurse is less likely to listen to the technologist. The nurse's dismissal of the technologist's questions compromised the safety of everyone in the room.

Some technologists employ methods to accommodate both the workplace hierarchy and the need to screen physicians and nurses. Such strategies acknowledge the authority of these individuals while still trying to keep patients and workers safe. A speaker at a conference I attended, who was a technologist, told a story that illustrates one method of accommodation. After apologizing to any nurses or doctors in the audience, she said, "I'll tell you how I deal with nurses and doctors, who are also a pain the ass. I'm passive aggressive so I say [she begins speaking in a sugary sweet voice], 'Okay. Let's split the difference. You leave the scissors and stethoscope here, and you can take your credit cards and watch into the magnet.' "[7]

The hierarchy between doctors and technologists is even pronounced in resident–technologist interactions, a potential site for hierarchical reversal since residents have little or no experience working with MRI. One site I observed trained residents. The technologists who worked at that site explained to me that residents, due to their lack of experience, were

---

[7] Credit cards will be erased and watches damaged by the magnetic field created by a superconducting magnet.

notorious for ordering unnecessary or inappropriate tests. When I asked a technologist, "Who tells the residents that that's actually not correct. The radiologist or you guys?" she answered by saying, "It depends." She explained:

> The fellows and residents in radiology have sort of a closer bond [to technologists]. So you can say, "Well, do you really think that you need that? Do you want me to try this?" You know it usually works. They don't take it personally. But if it's from an outside referring doctor from like, internal medicine or the floors, they don't want to hear from you that that's not the appropriate test. It should come from another physician. So it depends on what type of resident. If it's a radiology resident, you're more comfortable. If you say, "No, you're trying to help them because the attending won't kill them for doing that." So it's different than a resident coming from the ED [emergency department] ordering all these tests.

The technologist feels comfortable confronting radiology residents in comparison to residents from other departments, but the interactions between them cannot overcome the hierarchical relations that build from the two professions. Even with radiology residents, who were still in a process of training, the technologist never directly contradicted the residents. She changed their opinion through deferential questions that keep both the authority and ultimate decisions in the hands of the residents. Referring to the potential wrath of the attending physician further secures compliance from the resident and reaffirms the prevailing authority of physicians.

Economic, Social, and Physical Distances

Economic, social, and physical distances all contribute to the working hierarchy of an imaging unit. Income differences between radiologists and technologists are pronounced. In 2004, the median income for diagnostic radiologists was $364,899 (RSNA News 2005). The radiologists I interviewed suggested the income for radiologists is more varied than these statistics suggest. They explained that radiologists who own imaging centers can make anywhere from $300,000 starting salary to $800,000 per year as they become full partners in the center whereas radiologists who work at hospitals earn closer to $150,000 to $180,000 each year. Thus, full-time radiologists can earn anywhere between $150,000 and $800,000, which is significantly higher than full-time technologists' salaries.

In 2004, the median salary for technologists was $64,415 with states reporting some variation due in part to the cost of living expenses and the strength of labor movements (ASRT 2004, 51). Many of the technologists I observed also worked overtime, which can add anywhere from $100 to $10,000 per year, depending on how many extra hours are worked. Consequently, the lowest paid radiologists earn double what technologists earn, while the highest paid radiologists make ten to twelve times the annual salary of technologists.

The profound economic distance between the two professions is both caused and compounded by differences in cultural capital. Radiologists typically have more formal education than technologists. As noted earlier, radiologists complete four years of college, four years of medical school, plus a three-year residency in radiology. In contrast, technologists have a high school degree and may have completed a two-year radiologic technologist program. Although some technologists have completed a bachelor's degree, they are a minority (ASRT 2004, 127). Such differences create two distinct social worlds with accompanying diversity in leisure activities, neighborhoods, access to schools, and consumption choices (e.g., type of car, clothes, eyeglasses).

The distance between radiologists and technologists is further emphasized architecturally with physical space. Each occupation has its own area of work. The technologists work near and with the MRI machine. The radiologists work in the reading room where they interpret examinations. Although each ventures into the other's territory, individuals spend the majority of the working day in their own spaces.

The social and physical distance between the two groups became especially noticeable when I attended an MRI conference. Sales representatives for the pharmaceutical company that sponsored the conference invited some technologists, radiologists, and me to dinner. Although it was a small gathering, maybe twenty-five people, the radiologists and technologists formed distinct social groups. The radiologists and technologists chatted with members of their own profession and then sat with these same people for dinner. Few radiologists or technologists crossed the unspoken boundary to mix with members of the other profession.

The social, economic, and physical distances between the two groups are great, yet each is well aware of the other. In my fieldwork, each profession engaged in discussion of the other group when alone. The two areas primarily brought up by the radiologists were technologists' personalities and job performance. Some radiologists critically analyzed the character flaws of technologists while in the privacy of the reading room. One radiologist exemplified this practice when he said "What a flake," after the technologist delivered a film and left the reading room. Another time, a technologist left the reading room, and a radiologist stated, "He's so passive-aggressive. I am sick of dealing with ———." This type of quick negative evaluation was common in my fieldwork.

Radiologists also critically analyzed the work done by technologists when an examination was flawed. For example, one radiologist I observed was quick to blame technologists if an image came out poorly. Pointing toward lack of skills and bad decisions about image parameters, the radiologist thought a faulty image resulted from technologists' blunders. Yet if the image quality was excellent, this same doctor did not credit technologists. Instead, he said things like, "She just ran the protocol. She didn't do anything to produce the image," or "The technologist's contribution doesn't matter. It's not important." Other radiologists engaged in similar discussions. Verbal comments about technologists' poor workmanship were common whereas praise for their skill or choices was not. These comments can be read as a slip that admits what is typically unacknowledged: the highly skilled and valuable labor done by technologists. The interpretive work of radiologists always depends on the skills of technologists whose decisions create image quality. That is, radiologists produce better interpretations if technologists construct excellent images, whereas the production of low-quality images adversely affects the quality of interpretive work. Yet the importance of the technologists' work is seldom acknowledged. In my fieldwork, radiologists primarily recognized technologists' contributions when frustrated.

Of course, not all radiologists engaged in this type of discussion. A few of the radiologists I observed expressed sympathy toward the technologists and defended them from unwarranted criticism. In one case, the technologist followed the radiologist's written order and scanned a particular part of the brain. The written order turned out to be incorrect. Instead of taking responsibility for his request, the radiologist blamed the technologist. He said that the technologist did not check the patient's previous examination to determine the exact area of the brain to be scanned, therefore the technologist screwed up. Another radiologist countered the accusation by stating, "Part of the problem is the techs don't have enough time to check previous scans." He then suggested that it was up to radiologists to be clearer in their requests. This type of response was unusual in my fieldwork. Radiologists commonly vented irritation by talking about the technologists' inferior skills and difficult personalities.

When alone, technologists also talked about the radiologists. These conversations revolved around who was good to work for, who lacked patience, and who was in charge that day. This content related to their lower position in the hierarchical relation between the two groups. The radiologists have the power to evaluate and reprimand technologists, whereas the reverse is not true. As a result, technologists need to be able to predict the behavior of the radiologist. Negotiating the work day means taking the radiologist's personality into account, and the discussions I observed were used to develop strategies to do this.

The technologists I observed also developed slang that temporarily reversed the professional hierarchy between themselves and physicians. "Magnet starved" and "magnet panic" were two phrases used by technologists to discuss the anxiety physicians displayed when the MRI machine was not working. According to technologists, radiologists and referring physicians "freak out" when the machine is down. When I asked, "Why?" one technologist explained, "A lot of diagnostic skills have been lost to imaging technologies." Another said, "Liability. Docs need to cover their asses." While the pressure to produce revenue and efficiency also contribute to "magnet panic," the use of such terms allows technologists to laugh at superiors' behavior.

The hierarchy, distance, and at times antagonism between the technologists and the radiologists present one way of organizing interactions between the two groups. These dynamics ensure that each will see the other as opponents, not as members of the same stressed workforce. One radiologist called attention to this when he described the relation between the groups as one of "warring tribes." Instead of working together to challenge assembly-line models of work, the two groups remain distant. The hierarchy and separateness of the two occupations leave them on opposite sides of a vast divide.

Worker Safety

Metaphors of factory work such as long-term machine exposures, company scientists, and worker hierarchies are useful tools for thinking about safety in MRI units. Factory work has always been potentially dangerous, and safety is a constantly contested issue among management, scientists, and workers. Health care work is also potentially dangerous, and there are safety measures to protect medical professionals and patients. Such measures primarily focus on protection from immediate biohazards while potential long-term threats due to machine hazards are ignored. Radiation, the exception to this practice, has been accepted as hazardous by scientists and policy makers, and guidelines protect workers from exposure. Yet questions about another invisible force—exposure to magnetic fields—are often dismissed.

The divide between technologists and radiologists discussed in the previous section becomes pronounced when applied to the issue of worker safety in MRI units. Radiologists, who are higher in status than other workers and who participate directly in assembly-line knowledge production, have the scientific authority to dismiss worker safety claims. For these reasons, I call them manager-scientists—a hybrid position that combines aspects of management status with the authority granted to scientific credibility. As manager-scientists, radiologists have different perspectives on the effects of constant exposure to high magnetic fields than technologists, who work more closely with the machine and are not considered scientific experts.

For the technologists I observed and interviewed, it remains unclear whether MRI technology is safe. Technologists are constantly exposed to the magnetic field produced by superconducting magnets. These workers move in and out of the examination room where the strength of the magnetic field is highest and, despite shielding, the magnetic field stretches into the adjacent room where they operate the computer. Moreover, the magnetic field is always present even when the machine is not in use. Many technologists felt the technology was safe for short-term exposure but expressed concern about the long-term effects of working in a powerful magnetic field. One technologist, for example, noted, "I think that for the patient it is safe. Because the patient will be exposed to it for a short period of time—forty or fifty minutes. But I am really thinking of the people who are working in it. Who are working eight hours a day in a high field magnet." Or, as another technologist stated, "I have thought more about the safety of the workers because the magnet is never shut off." Most technologists, when asked about MRI safety, made statements like "The jury is out," or "I don't think it's been around long enough to know."

In contrast, the radiologists and referring physicians I interviewed and observed expressed conviction that exposure to the machine was safe. Responses to the question, "Do you think MRI is safe?" ranged from "Yes" to "Oh yeah. No doubt about it." One physician responded to the question by telling a joke. When asked about safety, he explained, "I often quote from that first radiology rotation when we were discussing grand rounds and they showed these [MRI] pictures there. I remember there was a fellow that talked to us about it. He said, 'As far as we know this is safe. Maybe in ten years all the radiology fellows will end up facing north.' I paraphrase that on occasion." The doctor's story effectively shuts down questions regarding safety issues and sends a clear message of off-limits to potential inquirers.

In my fieldwork and formal interviews, physicians repeatedly expressed confidence in the safety of the machine and did not address the concerns of the technologists. For these physicians, safety was a non-issue. Only one doctor of the twenty-eight I interviewed and the many more I observed expressed concern about safety. This neurologist's concern focused on the well-being of patients and potential problems such as malpractice issues, not the safety of technologists: "I hope it is [safe], obviously, because I order 1100 scans a year. Roughly. So, you know, I still just have a little concern that twenty years from now we'll uncover a problem with it that we don't know about it, and then we are going to have some huge problem induced by all of these scans we are doing on people."

Some of the technologists I interviewed thought that radiologists were not concerned about long-term exposure in part because they were not continually exposed to the static magnetic field. For example, one technologist noted, "The medical people, who are the radiologists, they are not really concerned about it, because they are working away from the magnet. It's the technologists who work with the magnet, and the technologist doesn't have the ability or the time to do research about it." Since some of the technologists I observed worked at a research hospital, it made sense for them to think of the radiologists as researchers *and* physicians. Pointing to the link between one's subject position and potential research interests, this technologist suggests it is unlikely that radiologists will be concerned about safety since they work far from the magnetic field.[8]

Physicians' perception of safety affects technologists who question the potential dangers of MRI technology. When technologists ask questions about safety, chief technologists and colleagues often refer them to radiologists, who are considered expert sources. If radiologists think the technology is safe, this is exactly what technologists will be told. As one technologist explained, "When I was first in MRI, I had spoken to this doctor about this. I asked about it while I was pregnant. And he said, 'You shouldn't worry about it.' " This type of dialogue was reported by other technologists I interviewed.

Most research evaluates short-term exposure to the machine in use—a condition most likely to be experienced by patients. Studies document that tissue heating and skin burns, changes in blood pressure, hearing

[8] A posting by Emanuel Kanal (2000), another scientist who generally follows the trend of emphasizing the safety of the technology, illustrates how one's location to the machine can shape perspectives on safety. A person wrote to Kanal's website and asked, "The magnetic lines running through my office will range form .1 Tesla (1000 Gauss) to .05 Tesla (500 Gauss). Is there any safety hazard?" In response, Kanal states, "There is no clear right or wrong answer to your question. If it would be possible to use another office without difficulty I would personally opt to do so." This response illustrates how a person's view can shift when they imagine themselves in a particular situation.

loss, peripheral muscle stimulation, and cognitive deterioration—all bio-
logical responses produced from short-term exposure to different components of MRI technology—do occur (see, e.g., Adair and Berglund 1986;
Brockway and Bream 1992; Ham et al. 1997). The research also shows
that, if managed correctly, many of these effects need not be a problem.

The focus on the patient renders the issue of long-term exposure invisible in the safety literature.[9] Even when long-term exposure, or the working conditions of technologists and researchers, is mentioned, it is usually
discussed in brief and generally positive terms. For example, John
Schenck's (2000) comprehensive review article focuses primarily on the
experience of the patient or short-term exposure. Because of this, positive
claims about safety, such as "there is good reason to believe in the inher-
ent safety of these procedures" (2, 15), represent the vast majority of the
text. The title of the article, "Safety of Strong, Static Magnetic Fields," also
highlights safety not risk, and this larger context sets a tone for how the information provided in the section on sustained exposure will be viewed.

Research scientists agree that there are three main areas of risk in regards
to MRI technology. They are (1) the external magnetic field created by the
main magnet in the machine; (2) the varying magnetic fields produced by
the gradient coils in the machine, which help make spatial information; and
(3) the electromagnetic radiation produced by the radio frequency waves.
Of the three potential areas of risk, the main concern for the technologists I
interviewed is the first because individuals who work closely with the technology are typically out of the examination room when the gradients and radio frequency waves are active. The technologists (or full-time researchers)
are exposed to a static magnetic field for the duration of their work day. The
strength of the field varies in relation to one's distance from the machine
and the actual field strength of the superconducting magnet.

Thus far, few studies have examined the effects of static magnetic fields
on technologists (see, e.g., Kanal et al. 1993; Tuschl 2000).[10] Although
these studies concluded exposure to MRI was safe, they were limited in

[9] The website MRISafety.com exemplifies this practice. The site, run by Frank Shellock, a recognized expert and prolific writer on MRI safety issues, is a valuable clearinghouse for risk
assessment and management. Nonetheless, the very design of the site negates long-term exposure as an issue: The link for "safety information" focuses solely on patient management,
and the link for screening forms contains only forms for immediate exposure. While this is
valuable information, there is no link for long-term exposure studies nor is there a section
dedicated to worker safety issues.

[10] In addition to conducting an extensive literature review, I consulted Carolyn Kaut, Frank
Shellock, and Emanuel Kanal, three writers who address safety issues, about long-term exposure studies. Kaut had heard of no such studies, and both Kanal and Shellock knew of only
their own study evaluating pregnancy outcome. I also contacted the American Registry of
Radiologic Technologists (ARRT). They also knew of no such studies.

scope. For example, Kanal et al.'s study examined the effects of static field exposure on pregnant workers. While MRI workers did have a slightly higher miscarriage rate when compared to homemakers, students, and other occupations, the difference was not significant by scientific standards. Kanal et al.'s study led to direct policy changes—pregnant women could now work through pregnancy—and helps support the physician's claim that the technologist shouldn't worry about exposure. Beyond Kanal et al. (1993) and Tuschl's (2000) work, there have been no longitudinal studies on worker exposure in general.[11]

Scientists and technologists interested in conducting further research on long-term exposure to MRI face significant barriers. New research draws on published literature and the perceptions created by it. In the case of MRI, the majority of research focuses on short-term exposure, which emphasizes the overall safety of the technology. This message is picked up by physicians, administrators, and the general public.

Here we see a well-known workplace scenario. Technologists, who are low in the pecking order, are concerned about the safety of long-term exposure to MRI and express doubts. Meanwhile, doctors and hospital management insist that MRI is a safe technology. This insistence occurs even though physicians primarily think of safety in terms of patients, not technologists, and scientific studies on the topic are rare and far from definitive.

The understanding of MRI as safe (and thus further research on occupational conditions as unnecessary) is bolstered by medical categories that classify technologies as either invasive (i.e., those that puncture or cut the skin) or noninvasive. MRI is considered noninvasive because the skin is not visibly breached, and this label is often evoked in information pamphlets and by health care providers as a way to justify the technique's lack of danger. Yet the radio frequency waves and magnetic fields created by MRI excite hydrogen nuclear spins to higher energy states during the exam thereby deeply interacting with the atoms of the body. As one technologist quipped, "Though MRI is officially categorized as a 'noninvasive' procedure, it

---

[11] A few technologists used the research done on exposure to the magnetic fields produced by power lines as a way to think about the risk involved in MRI. Such a comparison, however, is not considered "good science." First, the magnetic fields produced by power lines, although also measured in Gauss, reflect a different type of magnetic field than the type generated by superconducting magnets. The alternating current used in power lines create an alternating or varying magnetic field. In contrast, the magnetic field generated by the superconducting magnet creates a static or constant magnetic field. Second, the strength of the magnetic field created by power lines is much smaller (0.002–0.01 Gauss) than that generated by a high-field superconducting magnet (e.g., 15,000 Gauss for a 1.5 Tesla MRI system). For these reasons, many scientists think it is unsound to extrapolate from the data on the effects of power-line magnetic fields to think about technologists' exposure risks.

changes the polarity of every cell it exposes then changes it back. How 'non-invasive' is that!" This idea, as well as others, impedes investigation of long-term exposure to static magnetic fields.[12]

Combating the Dehumanization of the Workplace

The emphasis on productivity and volume in MRI units continues to intensify. Falling reimbursements from health insurance companies require MRI units to make up lost revenue by methods such as acceleration and specialization. Some innovative managers try to balance the pressure to increase volume with people's desire for variety and change. One manager, for example, insists that his technologists work in both CT and MRI units. He explains:

> If you notice, people who work longer in MRI, they hate working in MRI. If you go to any technologist who has been working for five or ten years in the MRI field, he is starting to hate the job. That's why I think that all centers must say, "You are working in CT and MRI," so that you can do the rotation. This has several advantages. One. The technologists will not get bored doing the same thing all of the time. Again and again. Two. They will stay in the field longer. They won't want to change the profession or the place they are working in.

For this manager, reducing employee turnover and fatigue outweighs the use of repetition as a way to organize work. Imagining a work environment that is simultaneously stimulating and productive, this manager insists on

[12] Despite barriers, there are avenues available to generate research on long-term exposure. First, technologists have two national organizations—the American Society of Radiologic Technologists (ASRT) and the American Registry of Radiologic Technologists (ARRT)—that could keep illness registries or sponsor long-term studies. The ARRT, in conjunction with the University of Minnesota School of Public Health and the National Institute of Cancer, investigates the health risks and conditions associated with technologists who perform techniques that involve long-term, repeated exposures to low-dose radiation. Initiated in 1982, the study tracks the incidence of diseases such as skin cancer and breast cancer in over 100,000 radiologic technologists. The ARRT or the ASRT could collaborate with epidemiologists to study the health effects of long-term exposure to magnetic fields. Second, technologists could dialogue with radiologists and other researchers about the risks involved with MRI to create new research projects. Collaboration between technologists and other scientists creates what Barbara Allen (2003) calls "citizen-situated science" or what Phil Brown and Edwin Mikkelsen (1990) call "popular epidemiology." Such approaches incorporate both the knowledge of citizens (or technologists) and the knowledge of scientists to produce science that is more fully dedicated to carefully evaluating neglected research questions.

rotating technologists through two different imaging techniques. His solution is unusual; most units emphasize gains in production without taking the vitality of workers into account.

The distance and hierarchy that exists between radiologists and technologists mean that it is unlikely these two groups will unite to challenge working conditions. Still, both radiologists and technologists make efforts, even if small, to bridge the divide. Why? Because the knowledge created through medical imaging is constituted in part by interactions between technologists and radiologists. The parties have a reciprocal relationship where communication is necessary: Radiologists write the initial request for the examination, and technologists translate the written request into concrete parameters; the quality of the radiologists' interpretation depends in part on the quality of the image produced by the technologists. If technologists and radiologists are upset at or distant from each other, both groups are less likely to communicate, clarify, and give constructive feedback on how to improve the production of the image and its interpretation. One technologist astutely tied it all together when she said, "Techs are people and docs are people, and you have to work together as a team to make things work. And it affects the patient care, and it affects the images, and it affects everything all the way down the line."

Individual radiologists and technologists try to cross the professional divide between the two occupations. But these efforts remain unsupported by the social organization of their work and broader categories of social class. Formal meetings between the two groups could facilitate alliances across these professional borders. Radiologists and technologists may talk between patient sessions, but there are seldom formalized meetings between the two groups.

"We are people too" was a frequent theme technologists and radiologists offered in interviews and in my fieldwork. "We are all human, and I think people forget that," said one radiologist. The need for technologists and physicians to call attention to their status as human beings speaks to the ways in which the organization of their work removes key components of identity (e.g., the desire to engage in varied tasks, express emotions, be spontaneous) from it. The emphasis on machinelike precision and reliability produces an efficient worker, one who is expected to repeat tasks and maximize volume. The radiologists and technologists I interviewed and observed resisted the trend by bringing creativity and care to their work. However, the stress on the rates of image production strained the limits of their endurance. Calling attention to the effects of the efficient workplace on workers' bodies and minds, a physician noted, "They are all tired at the end of the day. So much."

The assembly-line production process is not the only dehumanizing factor encountered by technologists and physicians. Patients seldom realize the constraints under which each group labors, and some of the health care workers I interviewed said that patients get impatient with them as a result. As one technologist explained, "We are limited in what we can do, and that creates a problem for us."

Chapter 5 moves beyond the actions of workers on the imaging shop floor to examine the marketing practices, health care policies, and other structural factors that create the flow of capital in the medical imaging marketplace.

The Political Economy of Magnetic Resonance Imaging

Magnetic resonance imaging, like all medical procedures, is a commodity that operates within political and economic systems of exchange. It represents multiple industries that generate income for the owners and producers of machines, parts, and accessories. Continuing to work with the concepts of commodities and mass production, this chapter maps the flow of capital in MRI manufacturing and service industries. Five factors—advertising, fee-for-service reimbursements, government investment and policies, medical standards of evaluation, and fear of litigation—operate in conjunction with cultural beliefs that link the image to transparency to co-produce the exchange of money in the visual medical marketplace.[1]

Attending to the corporate structure of medical knowledge illustrates how the growth and configuration of MRI industries are part of the economic transformations in U.S. health care that occurred during the 1980s and the 1990s. During this period, for-profit hospitals increased in number,

[1] Co-production theories call attention to the relations between science and society, and examine how each constitutes the other (Jasanoff 1995, 2006). In this framework, science is not a reflection of the social (defined primarily as political institutions), nor is the subjective nature of the social removed by science. Clarke et al. (2003) expand the co-production framework by theorizing the co-constitutive relations among culture, economic relations, state policies, technoscience, and actors. Their understanding of co-production complicates the definition of society, showing how it is comprised of many components—each of which is worthy of sustained attention.

replacing nonprofit institutions, and private companies owned and operated more areas of research, products, and services (Clarke et al. 2003; Turnbull 1996; Relman 1997a). As medicine moved toward a market model of health care delivery, patients became positioned as consumers. This was a time when advertisements for hospitals, drugs, and services proliferated, and the media told patients (now customers) to shop for the best treatment prices (i.e., ask for generic drugs, compare costs). The U.S. government even followed a consumer-choice model when it told seniors to evaluate and choose from a myriad of different Medicare plans for drug reimbursements.

To discuss the new economic and political dimensions of post-1980s biomedicine, sociologists Adele Clarke, Janet Shim, Laura Mamo, Jennifer Fosket, and Jennifer Fishman (2003) coined the term Biomedical TechnoService Complex, Inc. The concept, through the use of the words *techno* and *service*, highlights the shift toward a boutique model of health care delivery—one in which technologically produced information (and the resulting identities) are commodities for sale in a stratified marketplace. *Complex* and *Incorporated* denote the networks that resulted from the mergers and acquisition of hospitals, insurers, and pharmaceutical companies and the growing presence of private, multinational corporations in health care. They also signal the influence and significance of health care industries to the national economy, which represent "13 percent of the $10 trillion annual U.S. economy" (Clarke et al. 2003, 167).

As we will see, MRI–related industries are an important component of the Biomedical TechnoService Complex, Inc. The diffuse networks of industries and professions that produce and distribute MRI machines and examinations constitute a lucrative medical information industry—one that illustrates how anatomical images (and the knowledge produced through their use) can be understood only through analysis of corporate and consumer practices.

How Many MRI Examinations and Machines?

The number of MRI examinations performed in the United States and the income generated for multiple industries involved in MRI is quickly increasing. The IMV, a private research corporation, estimates that 21.9 million were performed in 2002 and 26.6 million procedures were performed in 2006 (Information Means Value [IMV] 2005, 2007). Industry analysts predict this number will continue to grow as new applications are found for the technology and it replaces computed tomography (CT) technology in some areas of body imaging.

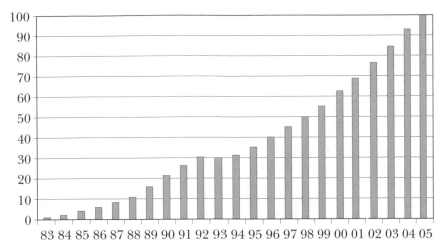

MRI utilization rates (expressed as the number of examinations per 1,000 of population) by year in the United States. Source: Robert Bell, *Decisions in Imaging Economics.*

In fact, total MRI usage rates have increased every year except for 1993 since the technology's introduction to clinical medicine in the early 1980s.[2] The health care debate in the first Clinton administration is thought to have slowed down MRI use in 1993 as physicians and health care professionals became more aware of possible scrutiny (Bell 2004).

MRI exams generate a constant stream of revenue for imaging centers, radiologists, and (as discussed below) a stream of revenue for the manufacturers of MRI machines. The following exchange highlights the revenue dimension of MRI:

[2] MRI–related industries have expanded and grown since the machine's introduction to clinical practice in the 1980s, yet data about the total number of MRI exams conducted each year are not readily available. State or national government organizations do not collect statistics about the total annual number of MRI exams or the number and availability of machines. Instead, for-profit and nonprofit organizations, such as Information Means Value (IMV) or European Magnetic Resonance Forum (EMRF), collect, distribute, and often sell such data. IMV, for example, sells its "2006 MRI Census" market summary report for $7,750; access to the entire 2006 MRI database is available for $65,000 (IMV 2007). The use of the word *census* links it to the U.S. census, a free, accessible public database that tracks information about people. However, IMV's database substitutes machines and exams for people and is for sale in the medical marketplace. IMV's appropriation of a word that Merriam-Webster defines as "a usually complete enumeration of a population; *specifically:* a periodic governmental enumeration of population" signals a broader social trend: the private ownership of knowledge. Occurring in many sectors of American life, including other aspects of biomedicine (Clarke et al. 2003), psychology (Schlosser 2002; Schor 2004), and technological and scientific research (Lessig 2005; Thackray 1998), the privatization of knowledge makes it harder for researchers, journalists, and the public to obtain data. Since information about imaging use is not readily accessible, various sources—both public and private—must be used in order to understand patterns in MRI use.

KJ: What are the first words that come to mind when you think of MRI?
Technologist: Noise.
Manager of the clinic: You know what I think of?
KJ: What?
Manager: Money.

An estimate of payments can be obtained from federal government data on the annual number of MRI exams through Medicaid and Medicare reimbursement statistics. The data is offered in raw counts for each reimbursement code. Calculating all MRI–related codes shows that the number of procedures submitted to Medicare steadily increased throughout the 1990s and 2000s, reaching over seven million in 2005. Annual payments for MRI procedures cost Medicare close to $1.75 billion in the same year. Medicare statistics represent approximately a sixth of the total number of MRI exams

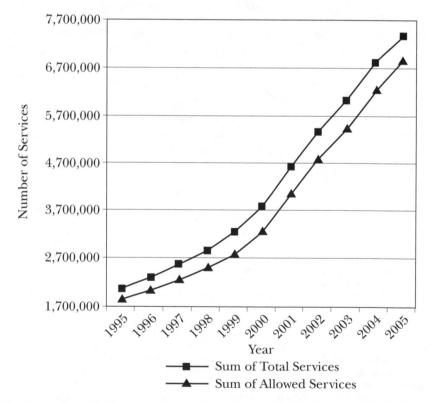

Total and allowed MRI services by year. *Source*: Centers for Medicare and Medicaid Services.

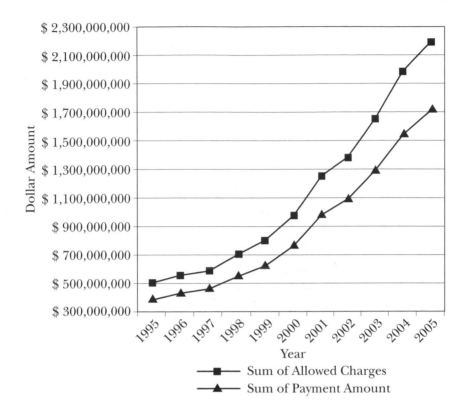

Allowed charges and payment amount for MRI procedures by year. *Source*: Centers for Medicare and Medicaid Services.

conducted each year. Thus, the total number of procedures and payment amounts are much larger than these figures.

The three sites I observed in my fieldwork were part of the national pattern of imaging growth. Two sites operated between three to five MRI machines and purchased one to three additional machines while I was there, which increased the total number of examinations conducted. The other site operated two state-of-the-art machines and kept the technology—both software and hardware—up to date. At all three sites, all machines were fully utilized. Empty slots were filled, and some machines were used twenty-four hours per day.

Lucrative Medicine: The Business of Medical Imaging

The expanding economies of MRI enroll an array of private companies, ranging from visualization technologies manufacturers to for-profit and nonprofit imaging centers and hospitals, and directly benefit certain medical professions such as radiologists. The business of medical imaging includes two levels of economic exchange: the manufacturing sector, which includes the production and sale of machines and other related products, and the service component, which includes the creation and interpretation of examinations. It is a lucrative health care venture that, at least in the current political and economic climate, guarantees a healthy stream of revenue for manufacturers, hospitals, and physicians.[3]

Level 1: The Production of Machines, Coils, Coolant, and Contrast

Estimates suggest that the United States had between 8,000 and 11,000 MRI systems in 2006 (European Magnetic Resonance Forum [EMRF] 2007; IMV 2007).[4] Transnational U.S., Dutch, German, and Japanese companies, such as General Electric (GE), Hitachi, Philips, Siemens, and Toshiba, control most of the medical imaging manufacturing market as well as the broader computer-based visual technologies sector. These corporations produce, market, and distribute MRI machines as well as other components of visual technology including televisions, DVD and VCR players, and video cameras. In breaking down cultural distinctions between entertainment/home media/private sphere and medicine/science/public sphere, corporations like GE, Hitachi, Philips, Siemens, and Toshiba manufacture and profit from the visualization of contemporary life.

Imaging centers in the United States currently pay manufacturers millions of dollars to purchase and install each MRI unit. Prices range according to the field strength of the magnet, the age of the machine, and machine design. For example, new 1.5 Tesla machines cost between 1.5 and 2 million dollars to purchase and install. Tesla is the unit used to measure the strength

---

[3] Centers could see a decrease in annual revenues if the demand for MRI exams does not keep up with the growth of imaging centers. A glut of imaging centers could saturate the market, ending the possibility of unlimited demand and twenty-four–hour service schedules.

[4] With the exception of Japan, other countries invest significantly less in MRI technology than the United States. For example, the United Kingdom operated 4.3 scanners and France had 2.7 machines per million population in 2003 (CIHI 2004). In contrast, the United States operated 19.5 machines per million population, whereas Japan had 35.3 scanners per million population in the same year. Despite the differences in investment, the United Kingdom and France are consistently ranked higher in health indicators such as life expectancy and infant mortality than the United States. (WHO 2006).

of an external magnetic field. Higher field strength systems have better spatial resolution and thus are considered more desirable. Open MRI machines generally have lower field strengths (e.g. 0.3 or 0.5 Tesla) and cost less. MRI machines with stronger field strengths of 3.0 Tesla represent a more significant financial investment with initial costs approaching approximately $2–2.5 million. Most clinical systems use machines that operate at field strengths of 1.0 or 1.5 Tesla (EMRF 2004; IMV 2007).

Besides acquiring the basic unit, imaging centers also must purchase coils, which are small pieces of equipment that enhance the content of the image produced. The price of coils can range from $10,000 to $90,000 each. *Cryogens*, another MRI–related product, are required to maintain the appropriate temperature needed by the magnet to function appropriately. Linde, Inc. (formerly BOC Gases), Praxair, Inc., and Air Products are some of the main companies that supply MRI cryogens. Hospitals and imaging centers negotiate multiyear contracts with either the original equipment manufacturer (e.g., GE, Siemens) or independent companies that subcontract with cryogen suppliers; the cost of contracts varies according to the availability of liquid helium, the main coolant used with MRI systems.

Another lucrative market has developed around the manufacture and sale of contrast agents. *Contrast* is a material that is injected into the patient; it illuminates the anatomical area being scanned, producing, as the name suggests, greater contrast between body parts.[5] Most MRI exams were initially conducted without contrast agents. However, approximately 45 percent of MRI procedures used contrast agents in 2006 (IMV 2007). Contrast agents represent a multi-million-dollar market (Medical and Healthcare Marketplace Guide 1998a, 1998b). Many companies (including machine manufacturers such as GE) develop and sell various contrast materials and even more want to get in on the act (Wolski 2006). Spending on MRI contrast media was approximately $342 million in 2003, and this market is expected to continue to grow (DeJohn 2005).

The use and promotion of contrast agents, coils, and other supplementary wares are an example of what is called *ancillary merchandising* in business. Ancillary merchandise ensures that even after the basic object is bought, customers will continue to invest in products and services. A clas-

---

[5] The use of contrast agents complicates the social construction of MRI technology as safe. A *contrast agent* is a material that is injected into patients and it can be (and often is) added to a routine MRI exam to enhance image quality. For most people these agents pose no significant health problems, but side effects can occur; e.g., General Electric's Omnivision can produce headaches, nausea, and dizziness. In rare cases, life-threatening anaphylactic or cardiovascular reactions occur (GE 2006). Contrast use therefore increases the riskiness of the technique itself since it adds an invasive procedure to the examination.

sic example of this common business strategy is the proliferation of Barbie products. By selling the Barbie, Fairytopia, Mermaidia, Bubble Vanity, Bath Vanity, Barbie Mini Kingdom Horse and Carriage, and other Barbie related merchandise, Mattel Inc. creates a steady flow of income for its company even after the initial purchase of a doll. Medical imaging companies, like many other industries including sport teams, media, and information technologies, use a similar business model. For example, in addition to the MRI machine, Hitachi also sells the QD Head Coil, the QD Flex Body Coil, and the Joint Coil. General Electric sells the contrast agent Omniscan as well as a range of coil technologies. While coils and contrast agents serve a purpose (i.e., they produce different kinds of MRI pictures), their sale simultaneously provides manufacturers with a continual revenue stream. Contrast agents, like the ink for your computer printer, must be replenished, and coils are perpetually updated and reworked so that new purchases are required to stay up-to-date.

With approximately 8,000–11,000 machines operating in the United States and that number constantly increasing, GE, Hitachi, Philips, Siemens, Toshiba, and other visual technology companies have access to a lucrative, expanding market, and a financial interest in the increase of MRI use. This financial interest is one driver in the annual increase in the number of MRI exams performed.

Level 2: The Production and Interpretation of MRI Exams

The second level of economic exchange is composed of the production and interpretation of MRI examinations. This level of exchange moves the discussion from manufacturing to the service sector of imaging, which includes hospitals, insurance companies, doctors, and patients.

MRI exams generate millions of dollars in revenue and are used to create diagnoses of health and illness for Americans with access to MRI technology. As noted above, approximately 27 million MRI exams are conducted each year in the United States, and this number continues to increase with no immediate end in sight (IMV 2007). In the United States, imaging centers and units charge per examination. A health insurance company may pay anywhere between $400 and $600 for a typical MRI exam without contrast agents—this amount is based on each company's unique negotiation of a contract with a site—and imaging units may do one to three exams per hour (Bell 2004; Poling 2004). The fee-for-service structure of imaging payment creates a financial incentive to produce more exams. As health economist Robert Bell notes, "To paraphrase the real estate dictum, the key to MRI financial viability is now volume, volume, volume" (Bell 2001, 1).

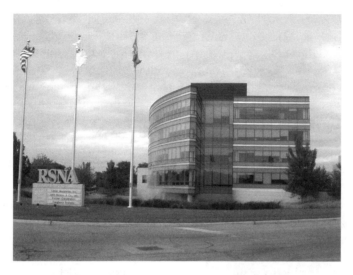

RSNA Headquarters building in Oak Brook, Illinois. *Source*: Radiological Society of North America.

Investment in MRI technology is expensive and requires considerable capital. Reimbursements, however, not only ultimately pay off the cost of equipment but also generate considerable income for the owners of an imaging facility afterward. The income goes directly into the pockets of owners, or, in the case of hospitals, it is used to offset other health care costs. The cost of contrast agents is now routinely added to the reimbursement fee for MRI exams, shifting the cost of using contrast agents from the MRI centers onto the insurance companies and patients. In fact, the use of contrast agents provides additional revenue for a hospital or center since they charge extra for its use.

Physicians benefit in this level of exchange. In addition to reimbursement fees for the exam and contrast agent, there is also a reading fee. This amount goes to the physician, usually a radiologist, who produces the written interpretation of an MRI exam. Demand for MRI exams is therefore also demand for radiologists' services. As noted in previous chapters, radiologists are among the best-paid physicians in biomedicine (AAMC 2005). The Radiological Society of North America recently announced that radiologists "are the highest paid players on the medical team," earning a similar median income if not more than other lucrative medical specialties such as cardiac surgeons (RSNA 2003).[6]

---

[6] Organizations that represent radiologists actively work to ensure that radiologists will be seen as the authorities of image interpretation thereby securing their participation in

For the physicians I interviewed—both radiologists and referring physicians who order MRI exams for their patients—the wealth associated with medical imaging was obvious. Early in my fieldwork, a radiologist said to me, "Do you know how much money radiologists make?" Not sure where the discussion was going, I asked, "How much do they make?" He then explained that radiologists who own their own imaging centers can make close to a million dollars a year while radiologists who work for private units can make anywhere between $200,000 and $800,000 per year. The doctor confirmed that financial exchange was a crucial element of MRI. If ignored, a robust understanding of medical imaging was impossible.

The doctor's attention to the financial was echoed by most of the physicians I interviewed and observed. For example, in a discussion about MRI exams one neurologist stated, "There are neurologists and radiologists in the private sector who are giving good service and making lots and lots of money." Neurologists make more money, this physician explained, because they are able to see more patients by ordering MRI scans instead of doing in-depth clinical examinations, while the radiologists make money by transforming anatomical scans into written reports. In a conversation about medical images, another doctor explained that MRI use was increasing "because it's lucrative." While clearly not the only reason it is used, the economic side of medical images is a key dimension.

The RSNA Annual Conference

The Radiological Society of North America's (RSNA) annual meeting makes the intertwining of capital and knowledge strikingly clear. Nearly 60,000 individuals attend the six-day conference, which is held each year in the largest convention center in the United States, McCormick Place. Located in Chicago, Illinois, the conference brings together professionals, companies, and research, as well as dollars for local businesses. According

---

imaging economies. For example, the American College of Radiology (ACR) publishes glossy "Ask" posters that show an earnest-looking person wearing a white coat and, to make her profession perfectly clear, a blue name tag that says, "Radiology Dr. Sheila Jones." Next to "Dr. Jones" are the words, "Is the doctor looking at your x-rays a radiologist?" The posters, which can be purchased by radiologists or administrators, teach patients to question who is interpreting their scans and are supposed to be displayed in waiting rooms at imaging centers and units. The ACR also publishes "Understanding Radiology" pamphlets, which explain how radiologists are rigorously trained to interpret anatomical pictures. The brochures were developed after ACR research "revealed that many Americans did not know that radiologists were physicians and did not readily identify a radiologist as 'their doctor' " (ACR 2006).

to an RSNA press release (2005c), "attendees will occupy nearly 22,324 hotel rooms on peak night, spread over 67 Chicago hotels," and "attendees will contribute nearly $112 million to Chicago's economy."

The conference itself is divided between an exhibition space dedicated to technological demonstrations and a series of conference rooms in which physicians and other scientists present research papers. A dazzling array of machines, displays, logos, and noise fill the exhibition space, which is comprised of two large rooms, each the size of a football field. The scene of the exhibition space can be viewed from above as higher floors have windows that allow one to look down on the displays. Bridges and tunnels connect the exhibition area to the research presentation rooms. Here, doors open into dimly lit rooms where suited men and women give PowerPoint presentations on new imaging applications and findings. With 112 meeting rooms available for research presentations, this area of the conference is also large in scale. One radiologist I interviewed captured both the intimate relationship between radiology and technology and the excitement generated by the conference when he noted, "When you walk into McCormick Place you realize the tremendous, the level of the marriage between medicine and technology. The scientific exhibits that the radiologists present are very impressive, but surely it's the technological exhibits that really grab you."

Large manufacturers such as GE and Siemens spend millions of dollars on floor shows and demonstrations. For example, at one meeting Siemens—a large home entertainment and medical technology company— used live actors pretending to be news reporters to introduce preproduced fictional news programs that broadcast the newest developments in medical imaging. Using microphones, the actors (as reporters) spoke loudly as they tried to draw individuals passing by into the demonstration. The GE exhibit included a sophisticated three-dimensional video that took viewers into the body where future directions in visualization, and disease identification and management, were demonstrated. At the same conference, Hitachi, another large entertainment and medical technology manufacturer, used science to pitch new products. In this case, actors, dressed as lab-coated scientists, explained the benefits of different MRI systems to people who stopped at the exhibit. Other exhibits relied on yet another common tactic in advertising—the use of highly sexualized women—to promote products. In these exhibits, scantily clad women introduced the advantages of each piece of equipment to viewers.

The surreal atmosphere created by interaction with fictional characters is further emphasized by the incorporation of actual medical imaging technologies into floor shows. Conference attendees walk through and around different visualization technologies as part of an exhibit experience. The sheer number of machines as well as their size (MRI, CT, and PET machines are large) and nearness (one can reach out and touch them) creates an awesome display of technology, science, and progress.

The selling of imaging technology and associated products takes place both within and outside of the boundaries of McCormick Place. Salespeople from medical imaging companies take radiologists and other attendees out for dinner and drinks, and at times rent hotel rooms for ongoing parties. These events are crucial to the promotion of MRI and other imaging techniques, and, although less visible than the exhibition displays, signal the marketing-medicine nexus that is central to imaging knowledge production.

The physicians I interviewed were well aware that the RSNA annual meeting cost millions of dollars and that much of the money was used to market new technologies to attendees. For example, one physician thought GE alone spent about seven million dollars on the annual meeting and others clearly knew that the major companies were there to promote new products. Exemplifying this awareness, a radiologist noted, "If there is any form of imaging that is on the market, it will be on display there: MRI units, MRI units in trucks, CTs in trucks, mammography units be it for the office, hospital, or mobile. There will be every single imaging hardware available to view and at the same time there will be the reps who will be taking you to dinner. Taking you to this museum program or that program. Trying to wine and dine you. Trying to get you to look at their equipment."

The Marketing of MRI

Selling Visualization

The networks between salespeople and radiologists at the RSNA annual meeting create a reciprocal form of marketing in which radiologists (and their professional organization RSNA) and salespeople actively participate in the buying and selling of visualization technologies and applications. The RSNA meeting is, after all, the main annual conference for the presentation of scientific papers on radiology, even as it serves simultaneously as an exposition space for GE, Siemens, and other manufacturers. Radiologists themselves pay to participate in the RSNA and willingly venture into the manufacturers' displays.

In turn, salespeople provide radiologists with a sense of belonging—one that ties their profession to cutting-edge knowledge production and prosperity. Throughout the RSNA conference, radiologists are shown new technologies and given free dinners and drinks. Through such interactions, manufacturers sell the idea of medical imaging in general as well as the products of particular manufacturers. While some radiologists resist these messages, the high number of state-of-the-art machines in the United States suggests that the majority accept them. Moreover, radiologists stand to gain financially from the purchase of MRI equipment and, as a profession, have little incentive to challenge the pro-visualization, pro-technology, pro-accessories message of marketers.

The reciprocity of marketing extends beyond the RSNA annual meeting to include daily work sites and regional conferences. Salespeople routinely visit imaging centers and hospitals. Free coffee mugs, pens, and lunches are integral to these visits, as are the relationships that are created in the process. The ties between a salesperson and a particular site ensure that radiologists and administrators will consider the company in future purchases. Salespeople also promote the ideas that the newest machines are necessary to provide high-quality care and, as expected, that their machines and products possess advantages in comparison to those of their competitors.

Radiologists actively participate in this marketing relation. Radiologists accept gifts and, more important, may also conduct research sponsored by manufacturing or contrast companies. Such research evaluates products (e.g., coils or contrast agents) or new applications (e.g., images of the breast or arteries) and can be presented at the RSNA or regional conferences that may even be sponsored by the manufacturer of the product itself. For example, Berlex Laboratories, a key producer of the contrast agent gadolinium, sponsors conferences on gadolinium use and finances some of the radiologists' research talks given at them. Presented as academic meetings, these gatherings are simultaneously a form of marketing. Critical evaluation is seldom part of the events, and the message to attendees is "use the technology or product."

Direct Marketing to Referring Physicians

The relationship between radiologists and salespeople represents the most substantial financial investment in visual marketing. The referring physician's office is the next biggest area of investment. Owners and administrators at imaging centers use marketing strategies to maintain and increase the number of patients sent to them by referring physicians. These centers particularly target the secretaries of referring physicians because they are the ones who schedule exams for patients.

Marketing to referring physicians and their administrative staff can take various forms. Most imaging centers simply provide promotional materials that explain the types of services offered. Others have begun marketing their services more aggressively, however, by providing incentives such as free meals and gift certificates. A manager of an MRI clinic expressed frustration about a competitor's use of incentives in an interview with me. One of her main competitors had just begun giving secretaries gift certificates at local restaurants if they sent patients to their imaging centers. Deeply concerned about the practice, the manager noted, "It turns medical imaging into a business built on incentives, instead of one built on [product] quality." The manager also wondered what the practice meant for her future budget. Would she have to increase her marketing budget to stay competitive with imaging centers that use incentives? The manager did not think this was a good use of her resources, but it might be necessary. The added expense would not increase revenue, but it might be needed so that the center could maintain the same level of volume.

There are no laws that regulate the use of marketing to gain referrals. Imaging centers are legally allowed to market to referring physicians and their staff as well as to offer incentives. Furthermore, there are no laws limiting how much imaging centers may spend on marketing or incentives. The only aspect of the referral relationship that is regulated is the practice of self-referrals. By law, physicians who own part of an imaging center are not allowed to refer patients to their organizations for examinations.

Marketing to Patients

In the 1990s the Food and Drug Administration (FDA) clarified regulations so that pharmaceutical companies could directly market to consumers on television and radio (Greider 2003).[7] Since then the visibility of drug commercials has steadily increased. However, the ubiquity of direct-to-consumer advertisements has yet to translate into imaging markets. Some hospitals and imaging centers do buy advertising time to court potential patients, but the majority do not. Instead, marketing to the public relies on more subtle forms of advertising. Such practices rely on product placement in venues not normally perceived as advertisements such as news stories and popular science exhibits (Berger 2003; McAllister 1995).

---

[7] The omnipresence of such advertisements provides fodder for stand-up comedians, who cannot resist poking fun at the messages of good living intertwined with discussions of chronic disease and drug side effects. For example, the "Living the Life I Want" Valtrex campaign equated having genital herpes with living a life of luxury. Not surprisingly, the idea that one should want to have a sexually transmitted illness in order to be hip, rich, and beautiful took heat from many comedians, including Jon Bowman, the longstanding opening act for Lewis Black.

One striking example of this type of marketing can be seen in the "Radiology: Medicine's New Vision" exhibit discussed in chapter 3. The RSNA, the Disney Imagineers, and other radiological organizations combined forces to create the $6 million Epcot display (Kaiser 2000). The exhibit ran for three years and approximately 600,000 people viewed the exhibit each year. Sponsors officially called the exhibit a "public information program" (RSNA 2000), but it is a form of marketing. The exhibit included no critical evaluation of medical imaging techniques or their use. Instead, it simplified the role of images in diagnostic work in an effort to enroll the public's support for the technologies. Furthermore, the RSNA administered surveys to exhibit viewers. The surveys asked questions about people's perception of radiology, providing important marketing information for the organization. A reporter for *Diagnostic Imaging*, a medical imaging trade journal noted, "An expected benefit of the RSNA's educational outreach is a change in the public perception of radiology and radiologists" (Kaiser 2000, 1). While the exhibit was presented as an "educational outreach," the point of the education—to create a positive image of radiology through narratives about imaging technologies and their use—was clear to industry insiders.

Prospective patients are also taught the MRI machine's value through news stories that celebrate the purchasing of new machines or the creation of new applications (see, e.g., Johnson 2004; Kerber 2005; Poling 2004). Tracking news articles about MRI through electronic search engines such as LexisNexis Academic demonstrates how the technology makes headlines whenever there is a change in machine design or another use for it is created. These accounts act like press releases for companies since the celebratory tone they often adopt blurs the line between information and marketing. Reports that focus directly on the technology disappear in between press release moments, resurfacing when there is a new application or purchase by a local hospital.

Stories that link sports stars' diagnoses and recoveries to its use also help legitimize MRI examinations in the public eye (see, e.g., Associated Press 2004; Battista 2002; Olney 2002). Such accounts often anthropomorphize the technology because they claim the MRI (not health care professionals) shows whether an athlete is healthy or not. They also teach the public that the technology is the technique of choice when the elite are injured. The implicit message in these "advertisements" is: It must be the best technique available if it is used with celebrity athletes.

The indirect selling of MRI through news stories and popular science exhibits helps create consumer demand. Many of the referring physicians I interviewed spoke about patients asking for MRI exams during an office visit. One doctor relayed a hypothetical dialogue with a patient to illustrate this trend:

> Patient: I want to have an MRI.
> Doctor: Well, why are you here? How can I help you?
> Patient: I just want an MRI.
> Doctor: Well, why?
> Patient: Well, I have these headaches.
> Doctor: Well, let's talk about these headaches. Where are they?
> Patient: Oh, right behind my nose. I get all stuffy. I cough a lot.
> Doctor: So that sounds like sinitus.
> Patient: Well, I think I have a brain tumor.
> [To me:] So, what do you do with those kinds of patients?

This physician chose to limit patient access to MRI but found it somewhat fruitless because people can usually find a doctor willing to order an examination.

Commenting on patient requests, another physician noted, "Sometimes patients come in wanting one [an MRI exam], even when you feel they shouldn't have one." When this happened, the physician explained to patients why they did not actually need an MRI and found that, for the most part, patients no longer demanded one after these conversations. Such discussions require time and patience on the part of the physician, and as these examples show, the outcome (no MRI/yes MRI) is not always guaranteed.

Although scientific exhibits and news stories are important techniques for the selling of medical imaging, they are far from the intensive advertising that could occur. Manufacturers and imaging centers could buy advertising space on television, radio, and in print media to promote the machine itself or particular imaging sites. Specific requests such as "I would rather have a General Electric examination than a Philips" or "I want my MRI at the——center" are the desired outcome of such marketing practices. Patient demand for particular brands has already been documented in relation to pharmaceutical requests (Abramson 2005). If competition between imaging centers or manufacturers increases, direct-to-consumer advertising may be used as a way to maintain revenue in the future.

Fee-for-Service Health Care

The marketing of MRI would be less successful if the United States did not have a fee-for-service billing and payment plan in a predominantly privatized health care system. While diverse plans and companies constitute what counts as health insurance in the United States, fee-for-service reimbursements comprise the major form of economic transactions. In such a model, health insurance companies (or patients if they are uninsured or underinsured) are charged and pay for each service (i.e. each test, treatment, or consultation). This type of billing/payment strategy has two built-in incentives that help promote MRI use.

First, imaging centers are incentivized to perform as many examinations as possible because each one creates revenue. The revenue helps pay off the cost of the machine and eventually generates income for its owners. This inducement also supports the expansion of the technology to new uses and diseases. Sociologists Peter Conrad and Joseph Schneider (1992, 168) explain that the fee-for-service system "not only creates an incentive to provide more services but also to expand these medical services to new markets." In the case of MRI, new markets include using it to visualize areas of the body previously mapped by other imaging techniques (e.g., breasts, prostate glands) or disease categories (e.g., schizophrenia, attention deficit hyperactivity disorder) that have no imaging technology component at present. Thus, the payment structure of health care contributes directly to the trend toward medicalization.

Sociologists and anthropologists have a long history of investigating the increasing reliance on medicine to define and thus intervene in what is understood as normal and abnormal physical, mental, and emotional processes—a trend they call medicalization. First proposed by Irving Zola (1972), medicalization theory takes note of how, in the twentieth century, emotional, mental, and bodily processes such as depression, pregnancy, and sexuality have become defined as illnesses that require medical intervention and supervision. In addition, behaviors labeled deviant or criminal such as alcoholism get redefined as medical problems in need of medical solutions. Since Zola's groundbreaking essay, social scientists have investigated the creation of new disease categories such as hyperactivity in children (Conrad and Schneider 1992 [1980]), adult Attention Deficit Hyperactivity Disorder (Conrad 2007), and fibromyalgia (Barker 2005), as well as the increasing privatization and technoscientification of medicalization processes (Clarke et al. 2003). The search for new applications for existing technologies and thus new sources of income helps fuel the expansion of medical categories and techniques into all areas of life.

One of the neurologists I interviewed described the technology prolif-eration that is central to medicalization processes. His account shows how MRI use expands in two directions: (1) the technology is used to visualize more regions of the body (e.g., MR angiography), and (2) more tech-niques or what are called "sequences" in the industry allow the same part of the body to be imaged in different ways. "When I was a medical resi-dent, we didn't have MR at all for diagnostic imaging," he explained. "Then we had MR. Then we had MR angiography. When I was a neurology resident, that's what we had. We didn't have diffusion sequences. We didn't have susceptibility sequences, and we didn't have fat saturated se-quences." The neurologist, using a metaphor of propagation and fertility, concluded that MRI is "a very fruitful technology." While multiple factors, such as marketing and improvement in the technology itself, contribute to its "fruitfulness," the income created by billing and paying for each exam buttresses the desire to visualize the body in new and different ways.

Fee-for-service reimbursements have a second built-in incentive—one that financially rewards diagnostic clinicians such as physicians, nurse practitioners, and physician assistants who are able to shorten office visits and thus see more patients. This occurs because health insurance compa-nies typically pay the same fee for an office visit regardless of its length. As noted in chapter 4, the standard fee also tends to diminish over time. To-gether, these features—the flat fee-per-visit and the trend toward dimin-ishing reimbursements—create a financial incentive for clinicians to increase the number of patients seen in a given day because this increases their income.

This second incentive also has implications for MRI use. To compen-sate for shorter office visits, physicians must order diagnostic procedures, which include MRI exams as well as other imaging tests, blood tests, and the like, to come up with a diagnosis and treatment plan.[8] Moreover, or-dering laboratory and other diagnostic tests does not cost the health care provider any money because he or she bills a third-party payer (i.e., the in-surance company or the patient) for them. Thus, the two aspects of the

[8] The incentives of fee-for-service reimbursements also shape the practice and delivery of health care in Canada. In comparison to the United States, which does not guarantee health insurance for all citizens and has a mix of private and public insurers, Canada provides univer-sal coverage and has one insurance payer—the government—for most services. Despite these differences, studies show that Canadian health care professionals order the same number of many procedures (e.g., blood tests, x-rays) as U.S. doctors (Armstrong and Armstrong 1996, 39; Evans et al. 1998, 16–17). In some cases, Canadians actually order more services than their U.S. counterparts (Fuchs and Hahn 1998). Canada does, however, regulate the purchase of ex-pensive technologies such as MRI so these techniques are less likely to be ordered in Canada when compared to the United States.

fee-for-service system that work conjointly and are crucial to understanding current patterns of MRI use are the following: (1) fee-for-service payments encourage health care providers to shorten the clinical encounter to maintain or enhance their income, and (2) ordering diagnostic tests such as MRI examinations is a compensation strategy that does not typically cost the health care provider money or time.

Some of the radiologists and referring physicians I interviewed spoke about the predominance of fee-for-service reimbursement and its distinctive stimulus to order more procedures. One radiologist, who worked primarily with neurologists, explained that for some doctors:

> It's easier to write an order to have an MRI exam than it is to do a neurological examination [which is done in the physician's office]. Why spend 45 minutes with the patient when you can spend that same amount of time, see three or four patients, write the same order and charge the same amount per patient and make that much more income?

When income is tied to the number of patients seen, it is logical to use tests to create knowledge and to spend (here the economic meaning of *spend* is intentional) minimal time with each patient. In such a system, one physician explained, "time is money."

The bias toward ordering tests leads to a situation in which, as one physician noted, "the physician is more ready to order the study rather than examine the patients." Or, as another physician explained, "Doctors now are starting to treat MRIs versus the patient that is in front of them." As discussed in chapter 3, the problem with this practice is that it overlooks the fact that high-quality diagnoses result from evaluation of *multiple* sources of information. Among these sources, the clinical examination is both a resource and a starting place for prescribing and interpreting other tests.

Echoing a point of view I heard from most of the radiologists and referring physicians I interviewed, a doctor said, "Everybody gets a history and an examination. You need to go into doing the MR with a hypothesis about what you are going to find, so that you are not just shotgunning the situation and finding things that are not relevant to the clinical picture." A brief office visit does not provide the detail needed to create a robust "clinical picture." Nor does it provide enough time for the health care provider to fully mull over the intricacies of a patient's case.

A radiologist I interviewed expressed regret about the lack of value placed on the intellectual labor required to evaluate and compile the varied (and at times contradictory) output of diagnostic procedures. He noted:

I would prefer that there was some way that physicians could be compensated for thinking. We're only compensated for doing. And, really, thinking is the most important part. Time and again, when patients are surveyed, the thing they care about the most is that physicians thought carefully about their problem. But, unfortunately, that is the thing least valued by the insurance industry.

In a fee-for-service system, compensation for thinking would require payments to be based on the amount of time dedicated to a particular patient—either in the clinical encounter itself or for the physician's intellectual work as he or she processes the information culled from various sources. Since most health care providers receive a flat fee for each office visit or, in the case of radiology, for each examination interpreted, they are financially penalized if they take time to think about a person's situation instead of quickly moving cases through the clinical assembly line. For the majority of physicians I interviewed, the pressure to see more patients and think less was not a positive direction for health care. They expressed concern for physicians who work under such constraints and for patients whose quality of care is compromised.

Challenging Fee-for-Service Reimbursements

There are two main challenges to the hegemony of the fee-for-service system and its built-in incentive to use more technology. First is the move toward global payments (e.g., a set amount per diagnosis) for inpatient service at hospitals. Global payments give one payment per patient regardless of the number of procedures performed and have been adopted by some insurance companies. The second challenge comes from some forms of health maintenance organizations (HMOs). Beginning in the 1970s, health care administrators tried to control costs by having the same company (an HMO) provide health insurance payments and the delivery of care (i.e., conduct patient examinations and administer and process laboratory results). There is thus little financial incentive to order tests or services since the providers and insurers are under the umbrella of the same corporation and cannot put the financial burden of reimbursement on a third party. However, even this kind of HMO still refers out for complicated, expensive procedures such as MRI examinations as they do not typically own and operate their own machines.

Building on the spirit of these reforms, one possible alternative to the unintentional effects of fee-for-service reimbursements is to replace it with a system of global payments: that is, a fee-per-diagnosis rather than a fee-for-service system. Such a shift would decrease the motivation to order tests since the money received would have to be divided among all of the procedures ordered. "When health care providers get paid per patient, rather than per act, the financial incentive is to do as little as possible," explains medical journalist Lynn Payer (1996 [1988], xv). A fee-per-person reimbursement system would also diminish the profitability of producing imaging examinations (and other services) because the revenue received for creating them would decrease. MRI use is increasing, said one radiologist I interviewed, because it "makes money. But, if people have no reimbursement for MRI, you can see the drop like . . . [She moved her hand from shoulder height down lower to signal the downward slope of use]." Discussions about moving to global payments for all patients (both in- and outpatients), however, have yet to result in changes in the structure of health care transactions. A transformation to fee-per-person reimbursements may bring about its own incentives (e.g., order fewer services) and problems (e.g., lack of adequate care). Until such a change, fee-for-service transactions and their built-in incentives will continue to fuel MRI use.

Of the two models, it may be that fee-for-service provides the best patient care. Although the built-in incentives mean that it is more likely that unnecessary tests will be ordered, at least the patient is assured of a certain standard of care. My point here is not to suggest that fee-for-service reimbursements in themselves are the root of the problem, but to show that they, like all billing and payment schemes, have economic and diagnostic effects. Moreover, there are few checks and balances that counter the stimuli of fee-for-service transactions. For the most part, advertising, laws, and medical standards—all key elements of health care—promote technology use and development. While there are efforts to evaluate and control procedure use, the predominant force in health care as with many sectors of the U.S. economy is toward expansion.

State and Federal Policies Promote MRI Use

In addition to the pro-growth incentives of marketing and fee-for-service reimbursement practices, the state intervenes directly to advance imaging technology use and the flow of capital in MRI industries. While the economic surge of the late 1990s provided both "the will to consume" and the capital needed by individuals and hospitals to invest in technology, government (in its various local and federal forms) remains a crucial player in the political economy of medical knowledge production. Government policies support imaging economies through three key activities: (1) the reinterpretation of Certificate of Need (CON) and Certificate of Public Need (COPN) policies, (2) reimbursement approval, and (3) investment in research for new applications. These three practices contribute to the economic boom experienced by MRI-related industries and professions and help ensure its future expansion.

Reinterpretation of Government Purchasing Restrictions

Throughout the 1990s, individual states directly enabled the MRI expansion project by relaxing CON and COPN laws that required government approval before MRI machines could be purchased. Initially put into place in the 1970s, CON and COPN policies sought to control spiraling health care costs, which were thought to be related to the oversupply and overuse of medical procedures (Blume 1992, 186). These laws required both private and public health care institutions to submit applications to the state explaining why they needed a big-ticket item (e.g., MRI or CT machines) or a new building project (e.g., new specialty units or new hospitals). State agencies then evaluated whether the technology or health care facility was required or not. Only after state approval could nonprofit and for-profit businesses purchase a costly technology or build a new unit or hospital. This type of legal intervention aims to balance profit-making motives with protection of the public good. With this aim, it shares similarities to zoning laws that restrict the location and size of businesses or liquor licenses that limit the number of businesses that can serve alcohol in a particular locale.

By the late 1990s, however, state priorities had changed. Protecting state and patient expenditures were no longer primary concerns, and the legislative focus shifted toward increasing the availability of machines. While some states kept their original review policies intact, the majority of states, responding in part to pressure by lobbyists for both hospitals and privately owned imaging centers, loosened or dismantled them. For example, Rhode Island and Massachusetts weakened state restrictions so that it was easier for hospitals and imaging centers to purchase and operate MRI machines. Not surprisingly, the number of machines in these two states increased dramatically after this policy change (Kowalczyk 2002). The state therefore partially relinquished its role as the arbiter of health care policy and purchases, allowing profit motives to more directly drive the adoption of MRI technology.

The relaxing of CON and COPN laws was part of a broader "deregulation" movement that gained momentum in the late 1970s and early 1980s when President Jimmy Carter signed the Airline Deregulation Act

(October 24, 1978) and the Staggers Rail Act (October 14, 1980).[9] These acts removed government controls from airline and rail companies, allowing these companies to determine prices, schedules, and routes (Gerston, Fraleigh, and Schwab 1988). By the late 1980s and 1990s, the deregulation bandwagon was rolling. Headlines announced the removal of government restrictions on gas, electric, and telecommunications industries, and lobbyists worked to dismantle rent-control policies in cities across the nation (Dao 1993; Ross 1993).[10] These changes removed government surveillance mechanisms from many industries and allowed the private sector to have more control in the setting of prices and the supply and distribution of goods.

Despite debates over the strengths and weaknesses of deregulation, the elimination of state and federal governments as arbitrators of public goods allows the influence of corporations and markets to increase. That is, government policies (through deregulation) support the profit-making motives of corporations instead of tempering them with legislation that aims to protect goods such as housing or health care from the volatility of markets. In the case of MRI, CON and COPN regulations tried to allocate expensive technologies based on medical need. The loosening of these laws meant that proof-of-need was no longer rigorously evaluated, and hospitals and imaging centers could purchase the number of machines they thought the market would support.

Medicare and Medicaid Reimbursement Policies

Deregulation was not the only legislative force behind the expansion of MRI availability and use. Federal and state governments also endorsed imaging growth through Medicare and Medicaid reimbursement policies. During the 1990s, for example, Medicare, a federal program, approved reimbursements for a range of procedures, including MRI examinations of

---

[9] The term *deregulation* is itself an important term in knowledge production. Its linguistic meaning implies a taking away of regulation; in reality, however, deregulation is typically a process of reworking previous legislation or creating new legislation. For example, when California removed price restrictions on wholesale energy prices in the 1990s, it simultaneously created another regulation that insisted energy must be bought and sold in the open market. The absence of regulations implied by "deregulation" buttresses the ideology of free markets, which suggests that laws and government are not allowed to participate in markets. Yet, as scholars such as Polanyi (2001 [1944]) have shown, there is no such thing as a market free of intervention because governments must enforce the laws of all trade—free market or otherwise.

[10] For a discussion of deregulation laws in the United States, see Eisner, Worsham, and Ringquist (2000, 35–57), Himmelberg (1994), and Mudambi (2003).

coronary arteries, MRI as a first choice of image for disc disease, and use of specialty coils to enhance anatomic detail (Centers for Medicare and Medicaid Services [CMS] 2006). During approximately the same period, Medicaid, jointly administered by the federal and state governments, covered established procedures such as MRI exams of the brain and spine as well as innovative techniques such as magnetic resonance angiography of blood vessels in the head and abdomen (see, e.g., Novello 2002; Sullivan 2000). Requiring Medicare and Medicaid reimbursements for such services helped legitimize the technology's use by sending a message to insurance companies, medical professionals, and patients that access to them is a feature of standard care.

Today, as new uses for MRI technology and other imaging technologies are created, new reimbursement requirements for these procedures are developed by federal programs. In general, any imaging application recognized by the FDA and/or accepted as sound medical practice will be covered by Medicare and Medicaid programs. For example, CMS recently expanded its reimbursement policy to pay for the use of positron emission tomography (PET) scans to diagnose and follow all types of cancers if the provider participates in either a PET clinical trial or submits data to the PET Registry. This decision, as Lisa Baird, the spokesperson for CTI Molecular Imaging, a company that makes PET machines, notes, "is something we have been hoping for forever. It's a big deal for us, and it's a first step toward broad coverage reimbursement" (Brass 2005, C1). For CTI Molecular Imaging, Medicare and Medicaid reimbursements are an important "first step" because they may transform other health insurance companies' practices, leading to widespread reimbursement of new procedures and setting standards for fees. Even if other companies do not follow suit, Medicare and Medicaid coverage is a "big deal." Approximately eighty million people, a significant number of potential users of a technology, are enrolled in Medicare and Medicaid programs (Cebuhar 2006). This number is predicted to increase as more baby boomers reach retirement age.

The Government's Investment in New MRI Applications

Finally, the federal government, via the National Institutes of Health (NIH), promotes MRI use by investing in research that considers new applications of the technology. The explicit aim of this type of investment is to create knowledge that will aid diagnostic and treatment work in biomedical practice. Yet, when successful, such projects also produce new markets for MRI by expanding its use to new fields of medicine and disease categories. Three imaging initiatives—(1) The Human Brain Project, (2) the Decade of the Brain, and (3) the Alzheimer's Disease Neuroimaging Initiative (ADNI)—illustrate this third way that government agencies promote the expansion of MRI use. Since the effects of these projects are still unfolding, it is too soon to know which ones will have a lasting impact on imaging use and clinical practice.

The Human Brain Project

In 1993 the National Institute of Mental Health (NIMH) and four other government organizations launched the $14 million Human Brain Project, which aimed to construct a digital archive of brain images (NIMH 2002). The initiative involved numerous scientists and laboratories across the United States and Europe and included millions of dollars in additional funding obtained through private grants and other nations' contributions (Hotz 2001; Kahn 2001). MRI was fully established as a diagnostic technology in relation to cancer and muscle impairments by this time period, and the Human Brain Project offered the possibility of creating a visual database that could be used to study the diagnostic biomarkers and efficacy of treatments for a range of brain-related diseases. The project sought to provide the basic research needed to expand MRI use to new domains.

For the first part of the project, researchers used standard MRI technology to visualize brain anatomy. During its second phase, scientists enlisted functional MRI, commonly called fMRI, to investigate which parts of the brain are activated in different activities or diseases. A functional MRI exam measures changes in blood oxygen levels and creates a visual black and white representation of the brain in action.

The use of both techniques ensured that the archive would contain anatomical images as well as models of how the brain functions; that is, researchers used MRI scans to study structural changes in anatomy, while fMRI scans were used to investigate which brain functions are affected by different diseases or disorders. The inclusion of fMRI exams helped legitimize fMRI as a visualization technique and made it easier for researchers to work with both kinds of images in subsequent projects.

The Decade of the Brain

The Decade of the Brain, a major government initiative that spanned from 1990 through 1999, was sponsored by the Library of Congress and the NIMH. It occurred concurrently with the Human Brain Project, and some scientists and laboratories contributed to and drew on both projects. Topics addressed in the initiative included schizophrenia, depressive illnesses, anxiety disorders, and learning disorders. Visualization technologies were central to scientists' investigation of these disease categories (Library of Congress 2000). For example, during the 1990s the National Institute of Mental Health, National Institute of Child Health and Human Development, and the National Institute of Neurological Disorders and Stroke funded hundreds of studies that sought to investigate whether mental illnesses could be clearly visible in MRI and fMRI examinations (Computer Retrieval of Information on Scientific Projects [CRISP] 2005). These projects evaluated whether imaging use could be extended to psychiatry and psychology—two specialties that did not use MRI to assess patients at the time of the brain research.[11]

Thus far, research results have justified the expansion of MRI use to academic psychiatry and psychology, although not to its use in a clinical setting. Investigations into brain imaging assert that there are associations between patterns in visual pictures and a particular disease category when groups are compared, but they have not shown correlations between brain patterns and the presentation of a particular mental disorder or learning disability in an individual. For example, scientists believe they have found brain patterns in MRI examinations that are shared by schizophrenics as a group, but the patterns are not seen in a predictable way in individuals.[12] That is, certain individuals who are diagnosed as schizophrenic may not exhibit the visual brain anatomy associated with the disease, while other people may have the anatomical markers associated with schizophrenia but are otherwise normal. Similarly, the research on attention deficit hyperactivity disorder (ADHD) found differences between normal controls and experimental groups, but it did not provide the specificity required to validate MRI as an individual diagnostic tool (Anderson and Teicher 2003; Sanjiv and Thaden 2004). These findings expanded MRI use to academic psychology and psychiatry where professors now routinely use the machines in ongoing

[11] The Decade of the Brain research and the Human Brain Project could also expand markets for pharmaceutical companies and other treatment providers. The desire to find a visual diagnostic tool coincided with pharmaceutical companies' release of new drugs (e.g., Risperdal, Zyprexa, Clozaril, and Adderall) for the treatment of schizophrenia and ADHD. Ideally these treatments will alleviate people's suffering, but they also represent economic transactions. If the use of imaging technologies enrolls more individuals into mental health categories, then more people will need biomedical interventions, thus increasing the market for various treatments.

[12] For a thorough discussion of the epistemological assumptions of between-group comparisons, see Dumit (2004).

research projects. It did not, however, provide the results needed to convince insurance companies, doctors, and patients of the image's value as a diagnostic tool in clinical practice.

The lack of the technology's use in clinical psychiatry and psychology may change.[13] Despite the unreliability of visual biomarkers as predictors of particular mental disorders, pictures of the "schizophrenic" and "ADHD" brain are routinely included in psychology and medical textbooks and lectures (see, e.g., Bernstein and Nash 2001; Myers 2003; Plotnick 2001; Weiten 2003). In addition, researchers continue to refine their search for visual biomarkers of particular mental disorders. These practices, coupled with a new generation of medical professionals trained to interpret the body via images in diagnostic work, suggest that imaging techniques could be used to diagnose individual patients in the coming years. If this occurs, the Human Brain Project and the Decade of the Brain research—in addition to expanding MRI use to experimental psychiatry and psychology— will produce even more uses for scans in the upcoming decades.

Alzheimer's Disease Neuroimaging Initiative

The Alzheimer's Disease Neuroimaging Initiative (ADNI) evaluates whether MRI can be used as a diagnostic and assessment technique for people with Alzheimer's disease (Cahan and Dollemore 2004). The National Institute of Aging (NIA) is the primary sponsor of the $60 million, five-year venture, but government agencies such as the National Institute of Biomedical Imaging and Bioengineering Establishment (NIBIB) and the FDA and private sector organizations such as pharmaceutical companies also financially support it (NIA 2006). The partnership between the government and corporations is a shift from the format followed in the Decade of the Brain research where each group funded projects separately even though topics often shared the same focus.[14]

---

[13] I interviewed practicing psychiatrists, psychiatrists associated with university hospitals, and medical students to better understand the contemporary psychiatric field.

[14] The publicity for the Alzheimer's Disease Neuroimaging Initiative exemplifies the social construction of MRI as a lifesaving technique (discussed in chapter 3). For example, in one advertisement author and poet Dr. Maya Angelou notes, "I have friends and loved ones suffering from Alzheimer's. But I can imagine and hope for a world without this terrible disease. You can help make a difference. A major brain imaging study led by the National Institutes of Health may help us learn to stop the progression of Alzheimer's. Please consider joining the study if you are between 55 and 90." The ad, like other publicity materials for ADNI, solicits the public's support by combining the legitimacy of Dr. Angelou and the NIH with the idea that images can help create authoritative knowledge that saves lives and eradicates disease. The ad also shows how publicists for scientists participate in and produce common narratives about imaging. It is not simply journalists or television writers who misunderstand science and promote the narratives in their work.

The benefits of the ADNI research to patients are unclear at present. Diagnostic techniques already exist for Alzheimer's disease, and health care professionals already have ways to track whether a treatment is working or not. As I will discuss in more detail in the next section, medical standards require researchers to show that the anatomical patterns visualized in MRI exams are correlated with individuals diagnosed with the disease. Researchers do not have to compare the efficacy or cost of MRI scans to the efficacy or cost of established techniques (e.g., patient history, CT scans, diagnostic questionnaires) in order for it to become accepted as routine protocol. Thus, if research results justify MRI use as an assessment tool, ADNI will enroll a new group of users, Alzheimer's patients, for routine exams. The boon to MRI producers and manufacturers will be significant since an estimated 4.5 million people in the United States could potentially be diagnosed with Alzheimer's disease.

Taken as a whole, the three projects—the Human Brain Project, the Decade of the Brain, and the ADNI—illustrate the government's commitment to imaging innovation and expansion. In addition to these major initiatives, the NIH and other federal agencies sponsor research into the development and use of MRI techniques to visualize heart disease, breast cancer, and other illnesses and bodily processes. The government also funds the National Institute of Biomedical Imaging and Bioengineering Establishment (NIBIB).[15] The NIBIB provides grants to researchers who aim to develop new visualization techniques or accelerate the application of existing techniques to more areas of the body and diseases.

While the scientific and medical value of individual projects are debatable, it is clear that imaging initiatives create new markets even as they create new knowledge. With the creation of new information that solidifies and establishes disease categories, new markets are produced for imaging use as well as related products such as treatment interventions. The government's investment in new applications is further augmented by the private sector's investment in imaging expansion and use. Private foundations, manufacturing companies, and contrast companies all fund innovation studies.[16]

---

[15] The NIBIB's web address is http://www.nibib.nih.gov/. For a full listing of the National Institutes of Health, see http://www.nih.gov/icd/.

[16] The National Guide to Funding in Health lists funding opportunities sponsored by private foundations. Using the index, the grants dedicated to diagnostic imaging can be tracked. Review of the National Guide to Funding in Health (Falkenstein 2003) shows that the majority of diagnostic imaging grants were dedicated to the exploration of new applications. Only a few grants examined the efficacy of a particular imaging technique. The same pattern—an emphasis on innovation funding—occurs when company investment is reviewed.

Authors' disclosure statements in medical journals and conference proceedings make this fact clear. Such investments aim to develop new applications and techniques and, when successful, open the door for further expansion of imaging markets.

Definitions of Acceptable Evidence

The push toward expansion is further reinforced by legal and professional standards of technological evaluation. Such standards oblige physicians and researchers to show that use of a technology or procedure can do what is claimed in limited studies with a few patients. They do not have to perform clinical trials that show efficacy in a majority of a large number of patients nor do they have to compare it to older techniques to see which one is most effective for patients. While our health care system promotes the development and introduction of new technologies, this strength is not accompanied by a sustained effort to evaluate the efficacy of technologies before and after these technologies are introduced to clinical practice.

Former editor of the *Journal of the American Medical Association* (JAMA) George Lundberg (2000) tackled the issue head-on when he showed how a number of procedures—including coronary artery bypass grafts and bone marrow transplants for breast cancer patients—were used in routine medical care before undergoing a clinical trial or developing standards for their use. "The problem is that many new technologies are based on uncertain science. All too often good clinical trials are not conducted before a new technique is almost universally used and coverage is forced" (ibid., 9).[17] The concern here is twofold: First, technologies and procedures may be used that harm patients instead of assist them. Second, technologies and procedures may be overused thus creating higher health care costs for consumers and insurers.

In contrast to technologies and procedures such as surgeries, pharmaceuticals are under stricter scrutiny. FDA regulations require pharmaceutical companies to conduct four phases of clinical trials to evaluate a new drug, with each phase expanding the number of humans involved. The Phase III trials, considered the gold standard of evidence, are performed on large groups (i.e., 1,000–3,000) of human

---

[17] Social scientists also document how technologies and procedures are commonly used despite the absence of critical evaluation of their effectiveness (see, e.g., Guillemin and Holmstrom 1986; Timmermans 1999; Waitzkin 1997).

subjects, follow a standardized protocol, and are the last phase necessary for FDA approval. After a medication has been introduced to clinical practice, the FDA then asks for a Phase IV or postmarketing trial to determine a drug's risks, benefits, and optimal use in the general population.

Medical technologies and procedures are not evaluated in the same way. Although the FDA has moved toward more stringent guidelines for medical device approval, procedures and devices are not held to the same standards as pharmaceuticals (Merrill 1997). For example, large-scale assessment of efficacy is not required to create guidelines for a procedure's use. That is, biotechnology companies are not routinely asked to conduct large clinical trials that assess the relative benefit of new technologies by comparing them with existing ones nor are they required to conduct trials that evaluate the relation between a procedure's use and the health outcomes of patients. Other government agencies and health insurance companies also do not require this type of evidence for a procedure to be adopted as routine care. Thus, technologies and procedures can be incorporated into medical practice without in-depth assessment of their necessity or optimal use.

MRI and other imaging techniques—as diagnostic devices—are subject to similar standards of evaluation. In the case of MRI, the FDA requires manufacturers to demonstrate that each procedure visualizes the part of the body being scanned to a certain degree of accuracy. Manufacturers also have to provide detailed information about the algorithms used in software that scans the output of radiofrequency waves and other aspects of the MRI system that can affect the patient as well as supply other technical information (Center for Devices and Radiological Health [CDRH] 1998). Manufacturers do not have to demonstrate which protocols produce the best-quality images for the majority of people, nor do they have to compare the technique to preexisting ones in large clinical studies to show that it produces better results. In fact, the FDA does not regulate protocols, and individual institutions are free to decide which ones they will use. As discussed in chapter 3, the lack of regulation creates the potential for unnecessary or low-quality exams since both can generate increased revenue.

Beyond the FDA, there are no other government agencies that require efficacy or evaluation studies of health care procedures. The Agency for Healthcare Research and Quality (AHRQ) funds research that examines the cost, quality, and outcomes of health care. Other government agencies and NIH institutes also provide grants and contracts for efficacy and outcomes research.[18] However, this type of evaluation is not a required component of technology implementation as it is with pharmaceuticals. Moreover, evaluation research is severely underfunded in comparison to the billions of dollars dedicated to innovation studies (Lundberg 2000, 9). Biotechnology companies and medical professionals can therefore promote and expand the use of medical imaging technologies despite a deficiency of trials that evaluate whether the use of these products improves health or provides the most cost-effective, high-quality knowledge.

The government and health insurance companies' lack of emphasis on efficacy and outcome studies is beginning to be challenged by changes in medical culture. Until the 1990s, physicians and their key organizations (e.g., medical schools, medical journals, and professional organizations), emphasized research that showcased new techniques or extended the uses of existing procedures. For example, major journals such as *JAMA*, *Radiology*, and *Neurology* tended to publish articles that highlighted new uses for an established or new procedure instead of ones that evaluated a procedure's efficacy in comparison with other techniques.[19] Although there were exceptions to this trend, the *New England Journal of Medicine* being one, these exceptions were precisely that: exceptions. While some researchers undertook clinical trials that examined whether a procedure's use helped or harmed patients, and others compared two or more procedures to see which one was most effective, these projects were eclipsed by the attention paid to the promise of new technologies and applications.

During the 1990s the focus in medicine shifted from an innovation celebration to a discussion about the need for standards and better scientific evidence after escalating health care costs and restrictions imposed by health insurance companies captured the public's attention. Throughout the decade, news headlines broadcast how some health insurance companies tried to control rising costs by restricting patients' choice of doctors and limiting the number of procedures used (see, e.g., Hilzen-

---

[18] The Office of Technology Assessment (OTA) was a government office dedicated to the critical evaluation of a range of technologies. Founded in 1973, the OTA published reports on topics ranging from analysis of the effectiveness of selected prevention and treatment services for adolescent health issues to the evaluation of the health and safety issues related to aging nuclear power plants. After its closing in 1995, no institute or office was formed to take its place. The OTA provided an important site for evaluative work, but its work was limited by lack of mandatory review. As with current efforts, review occurred sporadically and was not required as it is with FDA approval of pharmaceuticals.

[19] I conducted an informal review of articles published in *JAMA*, *Neurology*, and *Radiology* to better understand the type of research articles published.

rath 1994; Palosky 1995). Decisions about procedure use did not seem to coincide with physicians' ideas of good medical care—a discrepancy that caused anxiety and anger among the public who were concerned about the quality of limited care administered in the face of insurance capitations. The Clinton administration turned the growing public concern into a social problem by using health care reform as a campaign promise and forming a task force to investigate avenues for change. Clinton's proposed reforms aimed to provide universal coverage, preserve patient choice of physicians, and reorganize the health insurance industry (Starr 1995).

In response to the heightened scrutiny of health care delivery and costs, physicians, through their professional organizations and publications, proposed their own suggestion for change: the creation and use of evidence-based medicine (EBM). Evidence-based medicine provided a response to the health care crisis that enabled physicians to ward off the threat of government intervention. It also addressed the increasing tendency of health insurance companies to interfere in clinical practice since it called for the creation and use of knowledge about the optimal uses for tests and procedures.

There are multiple definitions of *evidence-based medicine*, but most stress the development of clinical guidelines based on the best available evidence (McGibbon 1998; Sackett et al. 1996, 2000).[20] Within this paradigm, evidence is defined broadly, ranging from one's personal experience to controlled, randomized trials that evaluate a procedure's use. Evidence-based medicine thus emphasizes the need for standards and evaluation, and protocols are developed based on the best information available. The EBM movement calls for the production of high-quality research and for physicians to learn how to evaluate the strengths and weaknesses of various sampling techniques and research methodologies. Although interest in universal standards and the use of empirical research as evidence have been around since the 1880s, the term *evidence-based medicine* and the EBM movement did not gain momentum until the 1990s (Marks 1997, Timmermans and Berg 2003).

Radiologists at research institutions heeded the call for EBM, focusing in particular on the dimension of EBM that highlighted the production of large-scale assessment studies. Since journals, conferences, and medical training had previously concentrated on new technologies and new

---

[20] The School of Health and Related Research at the University of Sheffield has compiled a list of definitions of evidence-based medicine and their sources. The list is available at http://www.shef.ac.uk/scharr/ir/def.html.

applications for existing imaging techniques, practicing radiologists had to be taught why evaluation studies were of value. Researchers initially published articles such as "Why should radiologists be interested in technology assessment and outcomes research?" (Thornbury 1994) and presented papers on related topics at the Radiological Society of North America's annual conference to explain to colleagues why new definitions of evidence were needed. Such work asked radiologists to base their practice on good science (now defined as efficacy or comparative studies) and to be more concerned about the escalating costs of health care and the overuse of imaging techniques. The commitment to rigorous evaluation was further cemented when *Radiology*, a central journal for the field, added an "Evidence-based Practice" column in 2001 (Proto 2004).

Thus far, radiologists have conducted and published studies that compare MRI technology with other imaging technologies (e.g., CT; x-ray, and ultrasound) in diagnostic work. This research, although limited in scope, begins to create a nuanced view of the situations in which MRI provides the best diagnostic technique (see, e.g., Gaeta et al. 2005; Tsushima and Endo 2005; Ouwendijk et al. 2005). Such work aims to assess imaging use so that radiologists can simultaneously provide quality care and contain costs. However, four limitations prevent this research from transforming diagnostic decisions. First, the studies produced are few in number and produce a hodge-podge knowledge base where some conditions and uses get attention and the majority are ignored. Second, radiologists, as image experts, compare imaging techniques (see, e.g., Jarvik et al. 2003; Lim et al. 2005; Schram et al. 2004; Yu at al. 2005). They do not compare imaging technologies to other diagnostic techniques (e.g., blood tests, physical examinations, or diagnostic questionnaires). Comparison to nonvisual techniques is crucial to investigate when and where MRI use adds to the quality of patient care. Third, the results of assessment research are not disseminated in a routinized way to practicing radiologists and referring physicians. The research is available to medical professionals through publication in journals, but there are no institutions or networks that transform the knowledge into practice; that is, the research is published but little effort is made to carry the information from print to clinical practice. Finally, even if research parameters were extended to include nonimaging techniques and research results were distributed, factors such as fee-for-service reimbursement and direct and indirect marketing continue to fuel MRI use in biomedicine. Producing large-scale assessment of technologies may not be enough to counter the effects of these other components of visual economies.

Visual Testimony and the Specter of Litigation

The desire to avoid malpractice lawsuits is another factor in the political economy of MRI growth. The majority of physicians I interviewed believed that fear of litigation caused both them and their colleagues to order more MRI examinations. Because of the visual truth it seems to hold, MRI exams are ordered by doctors to verify their diagnoses even in cases where they are fairly certain about the cause of a person's problems. For example, one physician noted, "There is a component of defensive medicine. If you do the exam, you are less likely to get sued." Another doctor explained, "If I think the chance of error approaches zero, I will not do it [order an MRI scan]. But I do think there's a middle range where the liability issue scares me a little bit." In such cases, this doctor orders the scan to defend against possible court cases.

For the physicians I interviewed, the MRI exam works to reassure patients that they have received the best possible care (thus deferring a potential lawsuit) and, in a worst case scenario, can be offered as proof of diagnostic accuracy in court. The "risk of not looking," as one doctor put it, is too much for a profession concerned about malpractice issues. Discussing patients who are unlikely to benefit from an MRI examination, another doctor explained:

> We have a situation in which doctors do feel liable if they make errors of omission. There's no doubt that people do it [order MRI scans] to protect themselves. In situations like that, where people are pretty confident that there is nothing to find on an MR, it's that sort of patient. But they do the scan so they can have some sort of concrete documentation of that. Sort of self-protection. Whether they do it overtly for that reason, or whether they have just evolved into doing it partly for that reason, but without even being aware of it. I would think a lot of people must be doing it for that reason.

The doctor's perception of MRI scans as protection comes in part from their use as both symbols of quality care and evidence in the courts. Patients have used the decision not to order an MRI exam to support claims of substandard care in court cases (see e.g., Cranberg, Glick, and Sato 2007). They have also used examinations to support charges either of failure to diagnose or of misdiagnosis (see, e.g., Glick et al. 2005; Pierce 2006; Vidmar, MacKillop, and Lee 2006).

Doctors, through their own or colleagues' experiences as well as medical publications and news stories, are conscious of such cases. One doctor exemplified this awareness when he told the following story:

> If you have a patient that has a headache and your clinical judgment is that this is a tension type of headache, you treat it with the appropriate medication. The headache goes away. Fifteen years later the patient is found to have a brain tumor, and then all of a sudden thinks, "Well, I had the headache fifteen years ago. So why don't I go ahead and sue my doctor from that time. He didn't get an MRI scan on me." That's an extreme example. That's rare that things like that happen. [Laughs.] My chairman in [a city in the northeast] had something like that happen. A patient sued him like ten years after he saw him for some unrelated issue.

Beyond personal experience, some medical schools' curricula now include information about the perception of diagnostic tests in courtrooms (Brilla et al. 2006). Within this context, MRI is often named as a procedure that ensures legal protection. Thus, the status of the anatomical image as authoritative knowledge in popular culture and medical culture translates to the courts as well.

While the physicians I interviewed felt that doctors used MRI scans to protect themselves from and in lawsuits, the extent to which physicians do this nationwide is unclear because the topic has not been studied in depth. Most malpractice research focuses on physicians' perceptions of litigation, malpractice insurance, and their general actions taken to protect themselves from court cases. Studies show, for example, that physicians of many specialties believe that the threat of medical malpractice causes them to practice defensive medicine or what is more colloquially called "cover your ass" medicine (Klingman, Localio, and Sugarman 1996; Jacobson and Rosenquist 1996; Kachalia Choudhry, and Studdert 2005). In these studies, acts of defensive medicine were discussed in a general manner and included referring more patients to other physicians, ordering more tests and procedures, and avoiding risky patients. Moreover, studies suggest that physicians' *perception* of liability is more likely to influence ordering patterns than the actual likelihood of being sued (Elmore et al. 2005; Studdert et al. 2005).

In a notable study by David Studdert et al. (2005), 824 doctors were asked to list the specific acts of defensive medicine they used. The actions reported included the following: ordered MRI, CT, x-ray, or ultrasound for unlikely indications; ordered other tests that were not medically indicated; obtained biopsy regardless of other findings; referred patient to another physician in unnecessary circumstances; prescribed more drugs than medically necessary; and avoided seeing a high-risk patient. Of these, prescribing an imaging test was the most popular act of self-protection for all specialists interviewed except for obstetricians/gynecologists. For example, only 13 percent (11) of emergency physicians ordered nonimaging tests whereas 76 percent (63) of emergency physicians ordered a confirmatory imaging test. Similarly, radiologists and other specialists were more likely to order an imaging test than give a referral or ask for a nonimaging test or biopsy.

While more studies need to be done to see how common this pattern is, the data raises provocative questions about the relation between MRI use and the practice of defensive medicine. Ordering a scan is a plausible act of self-protection for several reasons. First, doctors (and patients) may believe it is one of the least harmful interventions available since it does not involve breaking the skin barrier as blood tests or other procedures might do. While this belief conceals the fact that imaging use can lead to unnecessary invasive procedures such as biopsies or surgery if the results are unclear, it often operates as a perceptual framework for the procedure as evidenced in its labeling as noninvasive and safe. Second, ordering an imaging test allows physicians to maintain their professional authority over a case since the results are sent back to them. Such control over a case would be lost if they referred the patient to another specialist. Finally, the cultural status of MRI exams both as evidence and as a symbol of quality care dovetails with doctors' sense that they must engage in defensive tactics. That is, the authority ascribed to MRI scans means that doctors are able to, as one doctor politely put it, "cover their butts" by ordering the tests.

In all, the three dimensions transform MRI into a technology of self-protection which, if ordered by the majority of physicians, would bolster examination use and thus the generation of capital in MRI–related industries. Doctors, lawyers, patients, judges, and jury members all participate in a cultural milieu that positions MRI as a form of visual testimony—one that is superior to other ways of picturing the body and that is crucial to negotiation of truth claims in a climate saturated with concern about malpractice issues. More research needs to be conducted, however, to understand the extent to which concern about litigation drives MRI use in the broader medical community.

A Marketer's Dream: Selling Images to Healthy People

Beyond ever-expanding clinical and legal uses, a new market for MRI and other imaging techniques is direct-to-consumer sites where consumers can directly purchase medical images without going through intermediaries. While the high cost and special safety considerations associated with MRI prevent it from moving easily into the shopping mall at the present time, it has moved into storefronts at high-end hotels in Japan and may soon expand to the U.S. marketplace. Other less expensive medical technologies such as ultrasound and CT have already moved into sites where physician referrals are unnecessary. Prenatal ultrasound facilities, such as Peek a Baby, Prenatal Peek, and Fetal Fotos, are in malls and stores across the country (Garza 2005, A1). Offering keepsake ultrasound photos, DVDs, and videos with accompanying musical soundtracks, fetal sonogram businesses are profitable and booming (Brand 2004). Enterprising physicians and business people have also brought CT scanners into shopping malls. Companies now offer body scans to consumers willing to pay out of pocket for them, and direct advertising to potential patients is beginning to occur (Barnard 2000, A1).

One business, the University MRI and Diagnostic Imaging Centers, is an example of direct-to-consumer imaging that simultaneously illustrates the status accorded to MRI in the broader culture. The company operates six imaging centers (all located in Florida). The centers showcase state-of-the-art General Electric imaging equipment and offer every type of imaging examination to members of the paying public, including CT body scans, sonograms, PET scans, x-rays, and MRI exams. Each is located in a freestanding building and some are in office parks. Of all the technologies in operation, the centers' name highlights only MRI. The name also exemplifies the blurring of boundaries between for-profit corporations and public or nonprofit institutions. Despite the fact that the centers are for-profit corporations, they call themselves a "university" and have links to government and nonprofit organizations such as the National Cancer Institute and the Alzheimer's Association on their website.[21]

The state's response to the move toward direct-to-consumer imaging both combats and permits it. The FDA challenges direct-to-consumer imaging establishments through information available on its website. For example, the FDA puts out a brochure called "Full Body CT Scans—What You Need to Know" that states that body scans provide "no proven benefits

---

[21] The University MRI and Diagnostic Imaging Centers website is http://www.universitymri .com/.

for healthy people" (FDA 2003). After emphasizing the value of CT to medical work, the brochure explains:

> Taking preventive action, finding unsuspected disease, uncovering problems while they are treatable, these all sound great, almost too good to be true! In fact, at this time the Food and Drug Administration (FDA) knows of no scientific evidence demonstrating that whole-body scanning of individuals without symptoms provides more benefit than harm to people being screened.

The harm arises when the anatomical findings on an image are unclear, and the doctor must pursue more invasive procedures such as surgery to determine that the ambiguous findings are the result of technical artifacts or normal anatomy, not a life-threatening illness. Despite the warning to consumers about the risks associated with the procedure and the lack of scientific evidence for its use, the brochure states that the FDA cannot regulate health care practitioners' promotion of full-body scan. The FDA therefore indirectly enables the move of imaging into the shopping mall by not demanding or having the power to control such establishments (Lewis 2001).

Unlike the FDA, state officials such as the attorney general have the authority to regulate shopping mall imaging, but they seldom use it. Limited resources combined with lack of licensure programs make it hard for state officials to regulate or control medical images in the marketplace (Garza 2005, A1). As the blurring of medicine and consumerism continues, the relation between government agencies and medical imaging will be crucial to examine. Given its restrictions and commitment to pro-visualization market actions, the government is not likely to intervene.

The widespread concern about chronic diseases such as cancer and multiple sclerosis joined by the moral imperative to take care of one's self creates an anxious, take-charge consumer who may be willing to pay out of pocket for pictures of his or her supposed health. While there are individuals who resist the increasing use of visual technologies, consumer demand for imaging techniques is steadily growing despite apprehension about their efficacy or purpose.[22] The presence of medical images in the mall and other

---

[22] Some companies also conduct a form of neuromarketing where they use fMRI to visualize people's preferences for products, policies, or politicians (McCarthy 2005; Wahlberg 2004). Such a scenario may sound like science fiction, but scientists are already working with fMRI to visualize one's thoughts and feelings (see, e.g., Ferber 2001; Graham 2005; Radford 2001), and this research has been picked up by a few companies who use the technology to visually evaluate people's perceptions.

for-profit businesses suggests that visualization techniques will be crucial to the performance of a range of technoscientific identities. Consumers can use medical images to define themselves as "normal" or "healthy." Much like photographs and home movies, consumers now also have the ability to use anatomical pictures to visually express their identities.

Rethinking the Role of the State

In the economies of imaging, money circulates from imaging centers to manufacturers, and from patients and insurance companies to imaging centers and physicians. With the turn toward storefront imaging, people can pay out of pocket for anatomical pictures of their inner bodies and selves. The exchange of currency in relation to MRI is co-produced by marketing, fee-for-service reimbursements, government policies, medical standards, and concern about litigation. Together, they create lucrative and growing imaging economies.

Government agencies and policies play a critical role in the formation of imaging economies. They legitimize and expand MRI use through deregulation, Medicaid and Medicare reimbursement practices, and research funding. In allowing the move of imaging from clinical practice to the shopping mall, the state indirectly sanctions direct-to-consumer marketing. The FDA, despite efforts to critique boutique imaging practices, does not have the mandate or resources to intervene in a substantive way and consequently allows the medical imaging marketplace to expand. While privatization and corporatization mark biomedical knowledge practices, the state still matters. Through both action and inaction, the government promotes a market model of health care.

In contrast to its bias toward private sector goals and agendas, government (in its local and federal forms) could intervene to create a more equitable distribution of resources. First, states could limit the number of for-profit imaging centers in operation. Since most state's Certificate of Need policies require evidence that a community needs health care services before businesses can provide them, these policies could be revitalized to restrict the number of for-profit imaging centers (Harris 2006). Some state governments are beginning to control the number of for-profit hospitals in operation by reviewing and limiting sales of nonprofit hospitals to for-profit corporations (Volunteer Trustees Foundation 2006). In a similar way, they could take control of the percentage of for-profit imaging businesses operating in health care by reviewing and limiting their creation.

Second, state or federal laws could require for-profit MRI centers to donate a percentage of their profits to Medicare or Medicaid or to a fund that provides free care to the uninsured and underinsured. Such policies would address the inequities of the current system in which the owners of private imaging centers keep the profit earned from producing MRI exams while hospitals use it to offset the cost of providing a full range of services to uninsured and insured patients. For example, in 2003 non-profit hospitals provided $23 billion in free care to the sick and injured and had to compensate for the cost of procedures not fully covered by insurance reimbursement prices (Bender 2004). Some states, like Massachusetts, already require hospitals to contribute money to public health care; such laws could be extended to include imaging centers as well. Given the current emphasis on free market capitalism, these changes are unlikely to occur without public pressure.

Corporate and government practices, reimbursement schemes, and medical standards all produce imaging economies. However, the selling of MRI would be far less successful if it did not tap into a cultural milieu that equates technologically produced pictures with truth, certainty, and identity. From picture-producing cell phones to DVD players and recorders, visualizing machines are central to the construction and performance of identities and relationships. Moreover, anatomical images, while challenged and debated, are often viewed as visual testimony—one that provides unmediated access to the body. While access to imaging techniques is stratified and uneven, the presence of the visual in contemporary life and the link between images and truth provide the technological support and cultural familiarity needed to legitimize MRI as a producer of techno-scientific knowledge and identities.

Analysis of MRI shows the dynamic reciprocity among technoscience, knowledge, culture, and economics always at work in biomedicine. Attention to the co-constitution of such processes is critical for analyzing products such as pharmaceuticals, home health care technologies (e.g., glucose monitors), and other medical techniques because each weaves together broader cultural conventions, economic exchange, and technoscientific support for individual and collective identities in complex and unique ways. In the case of MRI, the need of manufacturing companies and imaging centers to produce income, combined with the actions of government agencies, and a cultural and technical milieu that equates the visual with truth and identity, make anatomical images a sought-after commodity in an ever-expanding biomedical marketplace.

6

A Sacred Technology?

Theorizing Visual Knowledge
in the Twenty-first Century

Magnetic resonance imaging is a cultural icon. It evokes a sense of wonder among patients and medical professionals. Both the technology itself and the scans it produces serve as totems, or sacred objects (Durkheim 1995 [1913]). By offering the promise of definitive knowledge and health, these totems represent hopes and dreams. For physicians, MRI scans provide direction and a sense of assurance when exploring treatment options. As one neurologist I interviewed commented, "There are clearly cases right now that without MR, I would be shooting in the dark. MR provides me with the light to decide what path of a different therapy I am going to take." MRI is believed to provide a light as physicians travel along the often confusing, contradictory, and challenging medical path of diagnosis and treatment. Such light is needed to help clinicians negotiate the ambiguities of their work in a fast-paced, litigious environment.

Like their patients, physicians and technologists evoke the technology's sacred status when they discuss MRI through the use of words such as *miracle, awe,* and *magic.* One physician I interviewed explained that he feels a "thrill when he looks at MRI examinations." He further noted, "Ultrasound images are not aesthetically wonderful images, and x-rays cast shadows. So I think it's nothing short of a miracle to be able to look at [the body through MRI]." For another physician, MRI exams produce a sense of wonder: "I am still always in awe [when I see an MRI exam]; I stare at them for hours."

Still other technologists and physicians use language that aligns the technology with magic. When a resident watched the production of an image for the first time, she exclaimed, "MRI is a form of American witchcraft!" Another physician exemplified the link between the supernatural and MRI when he explained, "I have a theory that medicine has not evolved terribly much, sociologically, beyond the shamans. And, therefore, it's mostly magic. The more powerful the magic, the bigger drum, the better. When a patient is brought into a room with huge equipment for a long exam that has lots of noise and all sorts of bells and whistles, that's a much more powerful, potent magic than if a stethoscope is placed against the patient." For this physician, MRI is not simply a biomedical tool; it also represents a powerful form of contemporary magic.[1]

Patients also react to the machine in ways that recognize its technological and cultural power. Although most of the patients I observed during my fieldwork managed to complete the examination, some had emotional reactions to the machine. Fear and anxiety caused some to back out of the room or cry after they saw the machine. Other studies report similar responses (MacKenzie et al. 1995; Melendez and McCrank 1993), and the technologists I interviewed told me that this type of reaction occurs regularly. The stillness of the dimly lit, windowless examination room, the machine's large size, and the idea that this test might reveal whether one has an illness intensify a patient's emotional reaction to the pending procedure. Other imaging technologies such as ultrasound do not typically provoke similar responses.[2]

Situating the Image

Chapters 1 and 3 highlight how cultural beliefs about technologically produced images contribute to the power attributed to MRI. By investigating the emergence, perceptions, and uses of MRI in biomedical practice, this book reveals that this imaging technology can be understood only by looking at the economic, social, and cultural contexts that shape its meanings and uses. What counts as MRI varies as these contexts change. MRI tech-

[1] Advertisements for MRI on manufacturers' websites and in medical journals both draw on and reinforce the notion of the sacred. Bright, white light highlights the machine, illuminating the tube in the machine. Some ads place the machine in front of drapes, which further emphasizes the idea that these machines are beautiful objects. These techniques, both of which draw from sixteenth- and seventeenth-century European painting, create an aura of radiance around the machine (Berger 1973, 137–139).

[2] A patient does not have to go into the ultrasound machine to be scanned. Rather, the machine is positioned next to the patient, and the technologist puts a small wand, called a transducer, on the person's body.

nology and the knowledge it produces cannot be understood apart from these contexts; it is a "situated" knowledge (Haraway 1988).

Monica Casper's (1998) playful exploration of the multiple meanings of the verb "to culture" is useful for thinking about the symbolic meanings of medical procedures as well as the inseparability of science and culture. Emphasizing how culture is an *action*, Casper notes, "Usually the term culturing refers to growing a virus or other organic material in a laboratory. But it also captures the intensive activities and meanings that can congeal around a particular social object at certain historical moments" (17). Applying this definition of culture to fetal surgery, Casper shows how surgeons and other medical professionals simultaneously help construct and benefit from the idea of the personhood of the fetus. This idea helps legitimize fetal surgery and thereby contributes to its use.

Like this "culturing [of] the fetus" (Casper 1998, 16), there exists a "culturing of the image." Biomedicine activities, media representations, marketing language, and broader notions of photographic truth all contribute to the culturing of MRI scans. Biomedical practitioners and MRI manufacturers draw on cultural conventions and ideas about sight and knowledge to create a pictorial artifact that, in turn, evokes and contributes to broader understandings of documentary-style images as truth. Although the idea exists that images are posed and constructed, the belief that photographs provide an unmediated slice of the world remains salient (Berger 1973; Sontag 1990; van Dijck 2005). Given this myth of photographic truth (Sturken and Cartwright 2001), it is not surprising that the use and variations of MRI technology—like cells in a petri dish—are growing.

The myth of photographic truth is based on two key beliefs (Sturken and Cartwright 2001). First, the use of a machine to produce pictures is consequential. A hand-drawn picture does not convey the same sense of objectivity and authority as one that is produced by a machine (Daston and Galison 1992). Calling attention to the prestige attached to machines, a radiologist I interviewed noted, "Americans buy into a lot of the high-tech stuff." Or as another physician noted, "Americans love shiny new technology, and [MRI] happens to be that kind of thing right now." In the case of MRI, the ascription of certainty is heightened by the status attributed to large, expensive, complex technologies.

Second, the myth of photographic truth draws on the cultural belief that photographs reveal the physical world in an unmediated manner. With anatomical pictures as their final product, MRI examinations excite cultural ideas about photographs. Although technologists use MRI to measure quantitative changes in the body, the medical professionals I interviewed react to the pictorial component of the examinations. For example, one physician explained that when he looks at MRI scans, he thinks, "God, these pictures are beautiful." When I asked a radiologist to name his favorite modality, he answered, "In terms of pure aesthetic, like how pretty the pictures are, probably MR." A neurologist exemplified the tendency to use pictorial language when he explained that MRI scans represent the body "Exquisitely. Especially these flair sequences that we are using to paint beautiful pictures of the different substructures of the brain." These comments not only illustrate the propensity to highlight the visual component of anatomical scans. The use of words such as *beauty* and *exquisite* points to the exalted status of the image and shows how science is infused with religious language and meaning, positioning physicians themselves as artists or creators.

In a symbolic economy that suggests technologically produced pictures reveal truths about the body, MRI exams are viewed as a way for patients and clinicians to see what is really going on beneath the skin. This sense of techno-revelation adds to the excitement associated with scans. One radiologist captured this sentiment when she described her first visit to the Radiological Society of North America's annual meeting as "akin to being like Alice in Wonderland. I was wandering through the halls of this huge convention center, just seeing MRI pictures everywhere I went. It was like, my God . . . stepping into the body." Explaining the exhilaration MRI scans spark among clinicians and patients, another doctor suggested that the feeling comes from "looking at your own body. You just see the surface all of the time. But seeing what is inside is amazing." The use of science to produce the visual is, as one neurologist explained, part of the wonder. Discussing a brain scan, he noted that it was "exquisitely beautiful, because it was a face and head, and you could see the profile. It was a human face with the science inside it. And I thought that was wonderful—to be able to meld those two things together."

Yet despite their ability to awe patients and health care professionals with their beauty and promise of certainty, MRI scans can also cause sadness and grief. The physicians I interviewed were well aware of the power of images and used them carefully in patient care. For example, one physician explained, "We always talk to [patients] and feel them out for what they might want to see. We'll often just say, 'If you like, you can take a look at the images.' But, we never put them right up. Because a lot of people don't want to. A lot of people don't want to see things. They don't want things to be as graphic as all that." Another physician illustrated the idea that scans create a "graphic truth" when he noted, "Patients get a lot of relief from seeing the [MRI] study, even if it shows significant pathology. In effect, it gives them an explanation of what is going on." Or, as another physician explained, "I think in a lot of cases it's an impressive jolt to [patients] to see how abnormal the brain looks. How much of it is damaged and that sort of thing. That's actually why it's a sensitive situation." Physicians' reflections about whether to show the scans or not reveals the symbolic potency anatomical images hold. The meanings ascribed to the technological and the visual contribute to the sacred iconography of MRI as well as its authority as a producer of knowledge.

Follow the Users: MRI Exams as Work Practices

Drawing on science and technology studies scholarship, a central tenet of this book is that users matter (Oudshoorn and Pinch 2005). Following technologists, radiologists, and referring physicians in their daily work routine illustrated the dimensions of medical practice that help transform MRI technology into both the "right tool for the job" (Clarke and Fujimura 1992) and a cultural icon with symbolic value. Fee-for-service reimbursements, less time for patient–clinician interaction, the specter of litigation, the desire to practice quality medicine, consumer demand—all these factors contribute to the decision to use MRI exams in clinical practice. The relationship between manufacturers and physicians, which includes direct-to-physician advertising and stealth advertising in the form of academic conference sponsorship, also encourages the technology's use in clinical practice (Angell 2004). While contributions to diagnostic knowledge clearly play a role in imaging use, the analysis presented in the preceding pages shows that the decision to order MRI examinations cannot be explained solely by the logic of "it's the best" or "it's the most accurate" method of evaluation.

Observing physicians and technologists at work also allows us to untangle the relationships that exist between economics, institutional priorities, biomedicine, and cultural ideas and conventions. In the case of MRI, cultural meanings ascribed to technologically produced images work *in conjunction* with the institutional, economic, and political factors listed above. That is, the myth of photographic truth helps transform MRI into a technology of transparency. In turn, this symbolic meaning legitimizes the decision to use the technology in the face of declining allotments of time for clinical encounters, possible lawsuits, and the desire to practice good medicine. Such cultural ideas contribute to decisions in biomedical practice and policy making and help make MRI a highly desirable technique.

By focusing on the links between imaging use in clinical practice, corporate relationships, health care policies, and cultural contexts, *Magnetic*

Appeal moves academic analysis of medical imaging technologies into new sociocultural areas. Previous scholarship highlighted the culturing of medical images and the use of imaging technologies in research settings (Beaulieu 2000, 2002; Cartwright 1995, 1998; Dumit 2004; Hartouni 1997; Prasad 2005a, 2005b; Stabile 1993; Waldby 2000). Building on this work, *Magnetic Appeal* shifted the methodological focus to clinical practice and expanded the analytical terrain to include corporate relations and health care policies. Examining the linkages among economic relations, symbolic practices, health care policies, and clinical care shows how these realms shape and are shaped by each other, ultimately producing the desire for and use of medical procedures (Clarke et al. 2003).

Do Not Radiate (DNR): Efforts to Control Imaging Use

This book highlights how certain factors bolster the increasing use of MRI technology in clinical practice. From research funding, fee-for-service reimbursements, and indirect and direct advertising to an emphasis on speed and volume and the meanings commonly ascribed to anatomical pictures, the social scale is weighted to encourage MRI expansion and use. However, some medical professionals and policy makers are concerned about the increasing use of medical images and its effects on biomedical work. This concern can be seen in a joke told by people who work in clinical medicine. The joke reworks the medical instruction "Do Not Resuscitate" or "DNR," which refers to a written order from a doctor that informs medical staff that resuscitation should not be attempted if a person suffers cardiac or respiratory arrest; this is usually done when a person who is very old or who has a terminal illness wishes to have a more natural death without painful or invasive medical procedures. In the context of MRI and other imaging examinations, patients are encouraged to put a different DNR—one that stands for "Do Not Radiate"—in their advance directive. This new command alerts physicians not to order any more radiology examinations. As one radiologist explains, "The use of images is out of control. Even if the patients are dead, physicians still order radiology tests." Because of this overuse of MRI and other radiology procedures, the joke goes, "We are going to have to put 'D.N.R.' or 'Do Not Radiate' to get them to stop."

Health insurance companies, the Centers for Medicare and Medicaid Services (CMS), and some physicians engage in actions with that purpose in mind: to reduce MRI use. Two practices—declining reimbursement fees and the creation of evidence-based medicine (EBM)—aim to counter the otherwise overwhelming emphasis on expanding imaging use. First, as noted in chapter 4, insurance companies and CMS try to control the costs associated with increasing MRI use by lowering reimbursement rates. This tactic, however, often exacerbates the emphasis on speed and volume prevalent in health care work. Lowering the reimbursement fee increases the pressure on technologists and physicians to process more patients in a shorter amount of time to maintain the same level of revenue. It also makes the experience of being ill more challenging for patients as they are processed even faster through imaging assembly-line production processes.

Second, radiologists promote the creation and implementation of EBM as a way to control the use of imaging. Evidence-based medicine calls for the education of radiologists, providing them with the analytical skills they need to identify the strengths and weaknesses of research methodologies. Radiologists' interpretation of EBM also calls for the creation and completion of rigorous studies that evaluate whether the use of a particular imaging technology changes a diagnosis or alters the quality or quantity of life. Such studies might compare, for example, the accuracy of the information provided by MRI with the accuracy of the information provided by other clinical indicators used to diagnose a particular disease. Studies could also investigate whether using MRI changes the life expectancy for individuals who suffer from a particular disease. As chapter 5 notes, researchers have begun to compare the information gained from MRI exams with that produced by other imaging tests. However, little research compares the information provided by MRI with information created by nonimaging tests, nor is there research that examines whether MRI use changes health outcomes.

The promotion of these two dimensions of EBM—education about methodologies and the creation of evaluative research—represents an important intervention that may help physicians determine when to use MRI. Addressing a lack of training among physicians in research methodology may teach them to become more critical consumers of medical studies. The creation of evaluative research may also help policy makers, clinicians, and patients make decisions about imaging use with an eye toward providing quality health care.

The implementation of these two practices alone, however, is unlikely to curb the desire for and consumption of MRI exams. Physicians continue to use medical procedures and treatments even after well-designed studies show that they provide little or no additional benefit (Guillemin and Holmstrom 1999; Martin 1995; Payer 1996 [1988]; Timmermans 1999; Waitzkin 1997). Research suggests that various social factors—desire for profit, fee-for-service reimbursement system, and the American belief that doing something is better than doing nothing—contribute to the continuing use of technologies and procedures that have been shown to provide little benefit. Solutions intended to check the increasing use of medical images will, therefore, have to do more than produce evaluative studies. Simply changing research standards and questions will not be enough to challenge the desire for and overconsumption of medical procedures.

If members of the medical community or the public decide to address the growing and often unnecessary use of MRI in clinical care, their solutions will have to consider the structural and cultural factors that support this growth. Three practices in particular aid the growth of medical imaging: all three should simultaneously be addressed in further efforts to curb imaging use.

Changing the Fee-for-Service Payment System

First, the incentives created by the organization of the U.S. fee-for-service payment system need to be countered. As noted in chapter 5, the common use of a flat fee per office visit creates a financial incentive to shorten office visits. This reimbursement model encourages clinicians to order more tests in order to compensate for limited time with patients and protect themselves from malpractice suits. The fee-for-service system also encourages owners of imaging units (e.g., hospitals, radiologists, private imaging centers) to do as many exams as possible. Although laying out an alternative payment system requires in-depth analysis that is beyond the scope of this book, one possible solution is to modify the fee-for-service model. Modifications could include paying each doctor for the length of a clinical encounter instead of a flat fee. More rigorous evaluation of the clinical indications and geographic placement of MRI systems could be used to limit the number of exams ordered and the number of machines available. These modifications would encourage health care workers to spend more time with patients and use MRI less. There are many possible changes that could be made to alter the incentives of a fee-for-service payment system, but any solution to the challenge of overusing MRI and other procedures must consider the ways in which those who have the authority to order and deliver the procedure are compensated for that care.

Federal Oversight

Second, the U.S. government could require rigorous study of the efficacy of new procedures and tests as part of the review process. As noted previously, MRI was incorporated into U.S. health care with no comparative evaluation of how and when its use contributed to diagnostic work. Nor were studies conducted that evaluated whether its use helped produce better health outcomes for patients. Such federal requirements continue to be absent. Yet, there are many avenues available to implement formal review procedures.

For example, the FDA could build on existing policies and require such research. This type of legal requirement would address U.S. physicians' desire for evidence-based medicine and make it part of the standard review process. Such laws could require manufacturers to evaluate how MRI exams contribute to diagnostic work and patient recovery in order to receive FDA approval. Drug companies already have to perform efficacy studies as part of the approval and evaluation process. Requiring manufacturers of MRI procedures to meet the same requirements would thus build on existing laws and help create a body of knowledge that can help evaluate the use of medical imaging. In an effort to spur diffusion, the FDA could require manufacturers to submit such studies after the technological application is in use instead of prior to routine use. Alternatively, the Agency for Healthcare Research and Quality (AHRQ) could oversee evaluation of the clinical use of MRI procedures. There are thus multiple ways federal oversight could be implemented. A centralized system would not only mandate review of a procedure's impact on health but also it would make it easier for patients and clinicians to track down research.

Shifting Cultural Beliefs

Finally, if the use and perception of MRI are to be successfully contested, cultural beliefs about visualization and technology will also have to be addressed. As discussed in chapter 3, popular narratives tend to equate high-tech equipment with progress, and technologically produced anatomical images with authoritative knowledge. These perceptions encourage individuals to overestimate the value that imaging use has on patient care. As one physician noted, "We have oversold MRI. People that have an MRI think that all the answers will be found, but it can't do that." Part of the reason this technology can be oversold relates to the way it fits into preexisting cultural beliefs about images and technology. These perceptions will need to be addressed if those who pay for and deliver healthcare intend to challenge the demand for medical images.

The Role of Sight in Biomedical Knowledge Production

Cultural ideas that link sight to knowledge production not only shore up the status of MRI exams, but they can also blind us to other ways of knowing the body. As sociologist Jackie Stacey (1997, 57) explains, "The common sense of seeing, knowing, and naming in biomedicine is an acquired one. Its logic, however, is so familiar to many of us brought up in the biomedical culture that some detailing of alternative ways of seeing and, more importantly, ways of knowing seem necessary." The following three vignettes offer some ideas about alternative ways we come to know the body.

Smelling the Body?

Some researchers actively challenge the hegemony of sight and technology in biomedicine by researching the use of dogs and smell in diagnostic work. In 1989, a brief report in the medical journal *Lancet* described a situation in which a woman's dog kept sniffing at the same spot on her leg. The dog's repeated return to this area led this forty-four–year-old woman to ask for a biopsy. The diagnosis? Melanoma. The authors of the report note, "This dog may have saved her owner's life by prompting her to seek treatment when the lesion was still at a thin and curable stage" (Williams and Pembroke 1989, 734).

Building on this finding and other case reports, scientists have begun to investigate whether trained dogs can identify cancerous growths. Dr. Armand Cognetta, a dermatologist in Tallahassee, Florida, is one researcher investigating this topic (Neve 2004). Working collaboratively with dog trainer Duene Pickel, Cognetta evaluated a dog's ability to smell skin cancer. George, the dog in the study, found cancerous lesions on six out of seven patients, and, in one case, the dog sniffed out a mole that had previously been biopsied and diagnosed as benign. Other studies evaluate the use of trained dogs to sniff urine samples as a way to identify bladder cancer (Willis et al. 2004) and patients' breath to identify the presence of lung and breast cancer (McCullough et al. 2006). It is too soon to tell whether biodiagnostics, the use of trained animals to diagnose illness, will become a diagnostic technique in the future. The point here is not to suggest that trained canines can or should replace MRI technology. Rather, this vignette should prompt the question of whether alternative forms of knowing should be considered alongside technologically produced vision. In a society that values visual forms of knowledge production above all others, such an alternative may seem ridiculous.

Listening to the Patient's Self-Report

The clinical encounter, through its use of touch, sound, and sight and its emphasis on interpersonal communication, offers yet another way to understand disease. During an office visit, a clinician will ideally take a detailed patient history and conduct a physical or clinical exam, which can use touch (e.g., palpating the abdomen), sound (e.g., tapping the abdomen and listening to the resulting sounds), and sight (e.g., visual inspection of the patient's body). As discussed in chapter 3, popular narratives and reimbursement practices that devalue the patient history and physical exam need to be challenged. The following case study, told to me by the patient, illustrates that the clinical encounter remains a valuable tool in diagnostic work.

A seventy-year-old man with health insurance went to see his primary care doctor about recurring dizzy spells. His physician referred him to a neurologist, who ordered an MRI exam. The scans were interpreted as normal. At a loss to explain the dizziness, the neurologist told the patient that he could not help him. The symptoms, however, continued. After a few weeks, the man returned to his primary care physician in frustration. A more thorough discussion with his physician about recent changes in behavior caused the patient to realize that he had stopped taking his iron supplements. The physician followed up on this information by ordering a blood test for anemia. The test showed that the man's iron was lower than normal and probably the source of his recurring dizziness. A few weeks after taking iron supplements, the dizzy spells ceased. In this case, a conversation between the patient and clinician and the use of a blood test provided key information. If the conversation had occurred first, the MRI exam could have been avoided. Although MRI is a valuable diagnostic tool, the current emphasis on imaging should not blind us to the potential value of the information provided in the clinical encounter.

The Biochemical Body

Other medical professionals suggest that the stress on imaging technologies creates a biomedical blind spot that deflects research funds and attention from the pursuit of nonimaging diagnostic tests. For example, a 2006 announcement from the NIH's National Center for Research Resources showed that "imaging research centers across the U.S. will get more than half of nearly $22 million earmarked by the National Institutes of Health this year for grants to fund cutting-edge biomedical research equipment purchases" (Diagnostic Imaging Online [DIO] 2006). This money will be used to buy new technology that will foster new imaging applications and technologies. The bias toward anatomical pictures is especially salient when thinking about the prevalence of and concern about cancer rates in the United States.

Cancer is a highly publicized, common disease. People participate in breast cancer walks, twenty-four–hour Relay for Life marathons, and wear Lance Armstrong's yellow wrist bands to raise money for cancer research and show support for those who survive the disease. One of the ways medical professionals diagnose cancer is through imaging technology. For example, mammograms are used to screen for breast cancer, ultrasound scans are used to detect ovarian and other soft tissue cancers, and MRI exams are used to help diagnose brain and soft tissue cancers. However, some physicians and researchers are concerned that the emphasis on imaging detracts attention from techniques that would find cancer at earlier stages. Dr. Susan Love (quoted in Felner 1997, 42) exemplifies this point of view when she proclaims, "Imaging is not the answer. By the time you see cancer on a mammogram, it could have been there eight to ten years. And improving the imaging has improved the numbers by 1 percent, 2 percent, but it's not going to do it by 30 or 40 percent. What we need is a blood test or something that will find cancer very early on—in the first year or two."

In this quote, Love challenges the idea that creating more detailed pictures will result in meaningful changes in patient outcomes. Her concern about the direction of research is relevant. Should we continue to fine-tune images or fund research that investigates the efficacy of new tests? Research money and time are limited. Policymakers, scientists, and the public contribute to promoting the idea of visual knowledge when alternative methods of diagnosis might be more effective and less costly.

The Uncertainty of Health and Illness

We need to do more than challenge the hegemony of sight in medicine. We also need to examine the relationship between the desire for MRI exams, our cultural anxieties about highly publicized diseases such as cancer, multiple sclerosis (MS), and Parkinson's, and the uncertainty of clinical practice and illness. We are taught that medicine is a science—a systematic, logical enterprise that has standardized protocols for treating illnesses. As a result of these protocols, certain percentages of people get well whereas other percentages of people do not. The news media contribute to the belief that various protocols deliver positive results by celebrating medical success stories and innovations. Each medical breakthrough, discussed in conjunction with stories about science and percentages, promotes the idea that doctors can diagnose and treat illnesses with amazing certainty.

But medicine is an uncertain practice. There are many illnesses, such as Alzheimer's disease, MS, Parkinson's disease, and many cancers, that health care workers cannot cure. Moreover, there are bodily ailments that clinicians cannot diagnose. Not every disease will be "found" and labeled, and there are times when doctors, nurses, and physicians' assistants will simply say, "We don't know what's wrong with you." A doctor I interviewed illustrated the uncertainty of medicine when he noted, "The public expects 100 percent perfection. They don't expect [a doctor] to give them anything but a 100 percent black-and-white answer. But the problem with medicine [is that] it's an art and a science. It is sometimes gray, and there are not necessarily black-and-white answers. That's a problem for people to accept."

In the face of the uncertainty surrounding medical practice and a growing awareness of chronic, often untreatable diseases like MS and certain kinds of cancer, there is MRI—a technology to which the news media and television dramas ascribe certainty and authority. So it is not surprising that MRI technology holds great appeal. Imaging use offers a promise of certainty that assuages deeper concerns about illness and mortality, as well as whether medical care will deliver the results patients expect. But the question remains: Can medical imaging solve the challenges posed by chronic illnesses?

The historical record demonstrates that changes in the social and physical environment helped contribute to the decline in mortality rates of some diseases prevalent at the turn of the twentieth century. Research shows, for example, that medical interventions were not the primary reason mortality rates declined for individuals suffering from tuberculosis, measles, scarlet fever, or typhoid (McKeown et al. 1972; McKeown et al. 1975; McKinlay and McKinlay 1997). Instead, public health measures such as the provision of clean water and the use of sewer systems helped contribute to their decline, a fact that is often forgotten in popular accounts of these diseases.

Anxieties about cancer and other common diseases such as MS could be framed within this context. John McKinlay and Sonya McKinlay (1997, 21) support this suggestion:

> If one subscribes to the view that we are slowly but surely eliminating one disease after another because of medical interventions, then there may be little commitment to social change and even resistance to some reordering of priorities in medical expenditures. . . . But, if it can be shown convincingly and on commonly accepted grounds, that the major part of the decline in mortality is unrelated to medical care activities, then some commitment to social change and a reordering of priorities may ensue.

Although MRI and other medical imaging technologies can help clinicians diagnose and track the progress of a disease, combining biomedical interventions with an understanding of the social and environmental causes of disease may be the most effective route for good health.

Today, popular press reports often claim that "all imaging technologies are combining to allow us to see, to know, and to cure ourselves in ways unthinkable a century ago" (Dowling 1997, 56). Such claims foster the idea that imaging technologies will be our salvation (Haraway 1997). Manufacturers and publicists for physician organizations contribute to these narratives by selling MRI and other imaging techniques as truth-telling techniques that help restore health. Such stories encourage people who are anxious about the high rates of cancer to focus on medical imaging instead of directing their concerns toward changes in air quality, pesticide use, and other social issues that are believed to be connected to the prevalence of the disease (Honey 1995; Paulsen 1993; Arditti 1999). The attractiveness of imaging technology and the knowledge we think it holds should not deflect us from addressing matters that may have a more dramatic and real impact on our health.

The Other Side of MRI: Access and Stratification

The preceding chapters focus on MRI in clinical practice and examine the use of this technology within economic and symbolic systems of exchange. By looking at MRI *in practice*, the discussion in these chapters emphasizes the increasing use of medical imaging and the cultural, social, political, and economic factors that help fuel this trend. However, another side to medical imaging must be acknowledged. Even as the use of this technology in biomedical work increases, there are those who lack access to it.

The delivery and quality of health care in the United States is stratified. One's class, race, gender, age, and geographic location can shape access to cutting-edge techniques, and the quality of medical care varies across regions and centers (Institute of Medicine [IOM] 2002). Sociologist Alexandra Dundas Todd (1994, 12) discusses health care access disparities when writing about her son Drew's experiences during his treatment for a brain tumor. "What if Drew were uninsured or less privileged?" she asks. "Would he receive this level of care?" Todd's son was able to get high-quality care and treatment, which included an MRI exam, when he needed it because he had health insurance, connections, and people in his life who knew how to get the most out of the health care system. As Todd acknowledges, however, millions of Americans do not have access to quality care.

Few studies have examined patterns of access and exclusion to MRI technology (see, e.g., Carey and Garrett 1996). Previous research, however, demonstrates that access to expensive tests and treatments is influenced by demographic factors. For example, research on cardiac care has shown that race, gender, and ethnicity affect who gets referred for costly cardiac tests such as cardiac catheterization (Ford, Newman, and Deosaransing 2000; Lillie-Blanton, Rushing, and Ruiz 2002; Schulman et al. 1999), a procedure that involves inserting a catheter into a person's vein or artery, which is then pushed toward the heart. Physicians use the catheter to record the pressure and blood flow in the heart chambers; dye can also be injected to illuminate the vessels that supply the heart. Clinicians then use x-ray technology to see whether there are blockages. Women, African-Americans, and Latin-Americans are less likely to be referred to receive the procedure than are white male patients.

Fluctuations in access over time should also be studied. It is probable, for example, that the level of access to MRI varies with periods of economic growth and discussions of health care reform. Lack of access may increase in importance during periods of slow or depressed economic growth or during discussions of health care reform and cost-cutting measures. Indeed, if we examine the figures from the early 1990s when discussions of health care reform reverberated throughout the United States, we see that the number of MRI machines purchased and the number of scans performed decreased (National Electrical Manufacturers Association 1999; Hensley 1997).

It is also important to examine why MRI is affected by economic and social trends. Such shifts in use may be related to the negative side of otherwise positive media attention. Joe Dumit captures the press's interest in medical imaging in his interview with *Newsweek* science editor, Sharon Begley. When asked how she puts together science articles, Begley notes that "In the case of the PET [positron emission tomography] cover, there was a paper presented at the Society for Neuroscience [meeting]. It was just some interesting memory thing, for which they used a PET scan. The editors saw that and thought, 'Well, gee, the pictures are gorgeous. Maybe there's more that can be said about this.' So they started pulling papers and talking to people" (Dumit 1995, 93). Anatomical images catch the media's attention. Like medical professionals and patients, journalists are similarly captivated by pictures of the inner body.

The social context frequently shapes the tone of this attention. During times of economic growth, picture-producing technologies are often celebrated. Headlines and stories emphasize the positive aspects of these technologies (see, e.g., Cook 2001; Kirby 2001). Conversely, when the economy is stagnant or in a downward cycle, or when discussions about health care reform occur as they did during the Clinton administration, these machines may become demonized. They move from symbolizing all that is good about medicine to representing all its excesses (see, e.g., Hensley 1997; Weiss 1994).

Debates concerning the issue of access intensify during periods of decreased MRI use. As with the ordering of MRI scans, the decision *not* to order an MRI examination cannot be grounded in rigorous evidence because this type of research is rare. The decision to order or not to order an examination is made based on personal experience, work conditions, and social beliefs. This leaves individuals who have less access to MRI in an even more precarious position because it is likely that race, class, gender, and other axes of inequality will play greater roles in a clinician's decision whether to order scans.

Exquisite Images, Unruly Bodies

MRI must be understood within economic, social, and cultural contexts that shape views about and uses of this technology. In particular, we need to place the development and expansion of the imaging armamentarium in biomedicine within the proliferation of visual information in all areas of social life (Clarke 2004; Mirzoeff 1998; Stafford 1991; Sturken and Cartwright 2001). Technological innovations support the development of medical imaging, and cultural ideas about technologically produced pictures create a familiarity with MRI that catapults the technology into a highly desirable technique. The creation of biomedical images provides more visual artifacts for circulation, and this extensive and growing body of images fosters the idea that pictures are the appropriate medium for representing ourselves and our stories.

A physician I interviewed captured the importance of the visual and the link between media and medicine when he noted, "As we all know, a picture is worth a thousand words. All we need to do is turn on the television and see how appealing TV is. The visual media. It's much better at speaking to people."

Part of the reason MRI scans speak to people is because visual communication is an integral part of our daily lives. Images are ever present and represent a taken-for-granted way of understanding identity and social life. Popular beliefs that forge links between technologically produced images and authoritative knowledge also increase the desirability of anatomical pictures. To see is to know, and to see the inner body is to know one's disease. Or so we have been taught to believe. Although a useful medical technology, MRI cannot provide the objectivity attributed to it, nor can it—as a diagnostic tool—provide cures for disease. While its use may help some individuals in particular circumstances, it will not help everyone all the time. One physician called attention to this fact when he noted, "We have sold MRI as the panacea for everything, and this is not the case." As we are encouraged to move toward telemedicine or to have yearly body imaging scans, we may want to keep the questions and concerns this book has raised in mind. The promise of visibility is, perhaps, not as remarkable as it has been made to appear.

Appendix

Research Methodology

My analysis of MRI draws on in-depth research that includes interviews with four scientists recognized as developers of the technology, content analysis of popular culture narratives, fieldwork at three imaging sites and five MRI-related conferences, interviews with medical professionals affiliated with research sites, and targeted literature reviews. This multimethod approach allowed me to investigate how the history of MRI is told and to examine how health care policies, popular ideas about sight and knowledge, and changes in the organization of work practices co-create MRI in practice.

The Emergence of MRI Technology

To research the historical development of the technology, I conducted in-depth interviews with scientists who contributed to its invention and archival research. First, I interviewed Paul Lauterbur, Raymond Damadian, Larry Crooks, and John Mallard, four scientists involved in the creation of MRI technology, about design and data decisions made in the 1970s and 1980s. Each researcher was trained in a different scientific profession and was part of a different research site. Chemist Paul Lauterbur headed a laboratory at the State University of New York in Stony Brook, New York; physician Raymond Damadian directed the research laboratory at Downstate

Medical Center in New York; engineer Larry Crooks worked with the University of California at San Francisco research team; and physicist John Mallard led a laboratory at the University of Aberdeen in Scotland. While other scientists also contributed to the development of MRI technology, these four diverse researchers provide insight into the context and decisions that shaped early MRI research. I used open-ended questions to interview each scientist, and all interviews were tape-recorded and transcribed.

Second, I critically analyzed scientific papers and patents related to MRI, newspaper articles published during the 1970s and 1980s, and secondary historical accounts. These materials were used to understand the scientific innovations, political pressures, social actors, and social networks involved in the development of MRI technology. I also coded historical accounts for recurring themes and omissions. Examining how the creation of MRI is typically framed, I found that a sustained discussion of cultural contexts was often missing from standard histories. Analysis of both the archival materials and the in-depth interviews provide the data for the particular rewriting of the development of MRI technology I present in chapter 2.

Representations of MRI in Popular Culture

I examined the content of magazines, television shows, newspaper articles, popular science books, and museum exhibits produced between 1999 through 2006 to understand the symbolic meanings ascribed to MRI. Using Lexis Nexus Academic, I analyzed references to MRI in articles published in U.S. newspapers and magazines. I also read academic and popular books about medical imaging, viewed exhibits at museums and theme parks, and examined references to MRI in network television dramas. Friends, family members, and colleagues contributed to this component of data collection by keeping an eye out for imaging technology references in cartoons, television shows, and the like.

I used a modified grounded theory approach to systematically analyze how MRI was represented in documents and sources (Glaser and Strauss 1967; Strauss 1993). Using an inductive methodology, I read through articles, museum texts, and transcripts multiple times to see which narratives were commonly used to discuss MRI technology. After identifying key narrative frames, I methodically coded each document to see how often and when such frames were used. Since the social construction of a technology is an ever-changing process, future research should analyze emergent narrative practices. My findings apply solely to the years analyzed (1999–2006)—the narratives used to discuss MRI technology may change in upcoming years.

Ethnographic Research

The fieldwork component of my research occurred at multiple sites. To familiarize myself with new directions in imaging research and the professional worlds of radiologists and technologists, I conducted fieldwork at five MRI-related conferences: the Biomedical Imaging Symposium: Visualizing the Future of Biology and Medicine; the annual Radiological Society of North America (RSNA) conference; a Clinical Functional MRI conference; a Magnetic Resonance Angiography conference; and a conference aimed at preparing technologists for the state registry exam. During each conference, I took notes on presentation content. Presentation content included both the presentation itself and the question and answer period at the end of each presentation. I also observed how participants interacted with each other during and between presentations. Finally, I informally spoke with conference attendees during meals and between presentations. All of these observations were recorded in field notes.

In addition to this fieldwork, I conducted ethnographic research at three MRI units in the northeast. One imaging center was a freestanding clinic. Physicians and other health care professionals in private practice typically referred patients to this site. The other two units were located in urban, university-affiliated hospitals. These units worked with both inpatient and outpatient clients.

I gained access to the imaging sites through a variety of methods. Instructors at a Radiologic Technologist program helped me obtain permission to observe at one location. I got access to the second site by cold-calling the manager of the unit. The manager supported my research and helped me gain permission to observe at this site. Finally, after failed attempts to contact physicians and the office manager at a third site, a personal contact introduced me to a physician affiliated with the hospital. The physician then facilitated my ability to conduct fieldwork at this site.

I conducted fieldwork for approximately six months. Most of my observations were conducted during the busiest hours of the day, from 8 A.M. to 8 P.M.. However, I did observe a few overnight shifts. Due to heavy demand, many MRI units operate 24 hours a day. The overnight shifts are less hectic than the day shifts, and I found staying overnight in imaging units offered a different view into the work practices in the hospital, allowing me to observe a slower, more relaxed dynamic in units and to witness how technologists work with emergency cases (e.g., patients flown in from nearby towns and cities for diagnoses and care).

Each day I recorded my field notes while at a site. At night I reviewed and added to my notes. I also formulated clarification questions to pose the next day. For example, one day I observed a technologist adjust a component of the examination protocol. Later that night I realized that I did not understand why the technologist made that particular decision nor did I understand how the decision affected the images produced. The next day I asked a technologist about the action. Why would one make that decision? How did it affect an examination? Thus, I conducted fieldwork and analyzed field notes in an iterative manner—one that constantly evolved and changed as I experienced unit work practices (Barley 1990b).

The presence of a note-taking social scientist provided new opportunities for meaning-making. Although used to having other health care professionals observe their work (all three sites participated in educational exchanges with training programs, other hospitals, etc.), an observing social scientist was unusual. Confronted with this new situation, people made sense of my work in professionally specific ways. Many technologists asked if I was there to evaluate work efficiency. I made it clear that I was not hired by administrators. Rather, I wanted to understand how medical professionals use and think about MRI technology since it was such an important technology in popular culture and medicine in the United States.

In contrast to technologists, physicians were not concerned about possible evaluation. For the most part, the physicians I observed controlled their work practices and had no reason to think that I would evaluate them. Instead, they expressed curiosity about sociology; many wanted to know about the field, my research, and other sociological studies. They often discussed their undergraduate coursework and liberal arts education and used these reflections to understand my approach to medical technology. Over time, the technologists, staff, and physicians became used to my presence. Most assumed an educator role and patiently and generously explained technological, work, and professional issues to me.

Part of being accepted meant contributing to the functioning of imaging units. The number of machines, emergencies, and constant rescheduling of patients made the hospitals sites particularly hectic and in need of an extra set of hands. To help out, I occasionally answered phones, tracked down needed professionals, and spoke with patients if addressed. I never did physical labor (e.g., lift patients) that could harm myself or patients nor would I have been permitted to do so.

I built on the knowledge gained from these observations by conducting in-depth interviews with 48 technologists and physicians affiliated with the research sites. These included 20 interviews with technologists, 17 interviews with radiologists, and 11 interviews with neurologists. The gender and race of the 48 technologists and physicians interviewed were diverse to varying degrees. Of the 20 technologists I interviewed, 10 were men and

10 were women. Most technologists self-identified as white. One person identified as Asian-American and one identified as Latin-American. Of the 17 radiologists I interviewed, 14 were men and 3 were women. Most of these individuals also identified as white. Specifically, 11 radiologists identified as white, 4 radiologists identified as Asian-Americans, 1 identified as Latin-American, and 1 identified as African-American. Of the 11 neurologists, 10 were men and 1 was a woman. 8 neurologists identified as white, 2 identified as Asian-American, and 1 identified as African-American.

The gender and racial composition of this sample reflects national trends in each of these occupations. Nationally, MRI technologists are almost equally divided by sex. According to 2005 data, 61.6 percent (15,607) of the 25,563 technologists who renewed their American Society of Radiologic Technologists' registration and considered MRI either their primary or secondary sphere of employment were women; 38.5 percent (9,956) were men. Information on racial identification is not available for this profession.

As in my sample, radiologists are predominantly white men. The American Medical Association (2005, 9) reported that men make up 81 percent (26,130) of all radiologists, whereas women make up 19 percent (6,158). The race/ethnic identity of radiologists is primarily white. Of the 21,523 radiologists who reported race/ethnicity, 81 percent (17,501) identified as white, 11 percent (2,410) as Asian, 2 percent (411) as black, 3 percent (660) as Hispanic, 2.5 percent (530) as other, and 0.05% (11) as Native American.

Neurologists are also primarily white and male. According to the American Medical Association (2005), 77 percent (10,286) of neurologists are men, whereas only 23 percent (3,007) of neurologists are women. Of the 9,051 individuals who reported race, 74 percent (6,712) identified as white, 14 percent (1,227) identified as Asian, 5 percent (457) as Hispanic, 5 percent (490) as other, 2 percent (162) as black, and 0.03 percent (3) as Native American. These patterns are similar to the gender and racial composition of my sample.

Most interviews were tape-recorded and transcribed. Only one interview was not recorded. In this case, I took detailed notes on the respondent's answers. As with the content analysis component of the research, I used a modified grounded theory approach to data analysis; that is, I initially read through interview transcripts and field notes to identify reoccurring themes. I then systematically coded each document for a particular idea. In *Magnetic Appeal,* I highlight the common ideas and practices found in interviews and observations. I also signal divergent viewpoints whenever possible.

Targeted Literature Reviews

The knowledge gained by the interviews and the fieldwork was complemented by a review of medical literature. My interest in what counts as scientific evidence and the relation between "evidence" and imaging use led me to examine MRI-related studies published in medical journals during 1999 to 2006. I used the National Library of Medicine's electronic search engine PubMed/MEDLINE to investigate research that focused on medical applications of MRI. I also reviewed MRI-related articles published in *Radiology*, the *American Journal of Roetgenology*, the *Journal of Magnetic Resonance Imaging*, and *Neurology*. This targeted literature review allowed me to gain a deeper understanding of how biomedical professionals define evidence and how these definitions are debated and negotiated overtime. It also provided insight into what aspects of the technology biomedical professionals focus on and find valuable. For example, biomedical articles primarily concentrated on the promotion and evaluation of new applications (e.g., expanding MRI use to new body parts like the breast or new techniques such as functional MRI). Although critical evaluation of imaging procedures already in use is now an integral component of journal publications, this type of analysis is less common than evaluation of new applications.

The use of multiple research methods—content analysis, fieldwork, in-depth interviews, and targeted literature reviews—provide the data for the sociological analysis of MRI presented in this book. This methodological tactic shows the uses of medical imaging and the meanings ascribed to it can only be understood in relation to institutional, economic, and cultural contexts. Biomedical professionals and research scientists act neither as passive recipients nor as free agents. Instead, they help create MRI in practice even as their views of the technology are shaped by broader factors such as health care policies, changes in the organization of work practices, social constructions of the technology in the public sphere, and cultural views about sight and knowledge.

References

Abraham, John, and Julie Sheppard. 1999. "Complacent and Conflicting Scientific Expertise in British and American Drug Regulation: Clinical Risk Assessment of Triazolam." *Social Studies of Science* 29(6): 804–843.

Abramson, John. 2005. *Overdosed America: The Broken Promise of American Medicine.* New York: Harper Perennial.

Adair E. R, and L. G. Berglund. 1986. "On the Thermoregulatory Consequences of NMR Imaging." *Magnetic Resonance Imaging* 4:321–333.

Adler, Robert. 2003. "Inside the Damaged Brain: New Dynamic Techniques Provide a Deeper Look at Alzheimer's and Schizophrenia." *Boston Globe* (May 6): B14.

Allen, Barbara. 2003. *Uneasy Alchemy: Citizens and Experts in Louisiana's Chemical Corridor Dispute.* Cambridge, MA: MIT Press.

Ambrose, J. 1973. "Computerized Transverse Axial Scanning (Tomography): Part 2, Clinical Application." *British Journal of Radiology* 46:1023–1047.

American College of Radiology [ACR]. 2006. "Understanding Radiology." Retrieved December 1, 2006 (http://www.acr.org/s_acr/sec.asp?CID=1508&DID=15417).

American Medical Association [AMA]. 2004. "Medical Malpractice Reform—NOW!" Chicago: AMA.

American Registry of Radiologic Technologists [AART]. 2006. "R. T. Census by State and Modality." Retrieved February 23, 2006 (http://www.arrt.org/web/registration/rtcensus.htm).

American Society of Radiologic Technologists [ASRT]. 2004. *Radiologic Technologist Wage and Salary Survey 2004.* Albuquerque, NM: American Society of Radiologic Technologists Publications.

Anderson, Carl, and Martin Teicher. 2003. "Brain Imaging and the Diagnosis of ADHD." *Psychiatric Times* (September): 56–58.

Angell, Marcia. 2004. *The Truth about the Drug Companies: How They Deceive Us and What We Can Do about It.* New York: Random House.

Applegate, Kimberly, and Carol Rumack. 2003. "Workforce Problems and Strategies." *Imaging Economics.* Retrieved September 23, 2007 (http://www.imagingeconomics.com/issues/articles/2003-05_02.asp).

Arditti, Rita. 1999. "The Precautionary Principle: What It Is and Why Health Activists Should Embrace It." *Sojourner: The Women's Forum* (March): 14.

Armstrong, Pat, and Hugh Armstrong. 1996. *Wasting Away: The Undermining of Canadian Health Care.* New York: Oxford University Press.

Associated Press. 2004. "The Big Buzz Is Magnets: Once Rare, MRI Machines Have Become More Profitable." *San Antonio Express-News* (June 19): D1.

Association of American Medical Colleges [AAMC]. 2004. "Careers in Medicine: Specialty Information Radiology." Retrieved March 2005 (http://www.aamc.org/students/cim/pub_radiology.htm).

Axel, Leon. 2006. Personal correspondence, July 10.

Barger, M. Susan, and William White. 2000. *The Daguerreotype: Nineteenth-century Technology and Modern Science.* Baltimore: Johns Hopkins University Press.

Barker, Kristin. 2005. *The Fibromyalgia Story: Medical Authority and Women's Worlds of Pain.* Philadelphia: Temple University Press.

Barley, Stephen. 1986. "Technology as an Occasion for Structuring: Evidence from Observations of CT Scanners and the Social Order of Radiology Departments." *Administrative Science Quarterly* 31(1): 78–108.

———. 1990a. "The Alignment of Technology and Structure Through Roles and Networks," *Administrative Science Quarterly* 35(1): 61–103.

———. 1990b. "Images of Imaging: Notes on Doing Longitudinal Field Work." *Organization Science* 1(3): 220–247.

Barnard, Anne. 2000. "Clinics Market Scans for the Symptom-Free." *Boston Globe* (August 26): 1, A1.

Battista, Judy. 2002. "MRI Reveals Partial Tear in Abraham's Left Knee." *New York Times* (August 6): D1.

Beam, C. M., P. M. Layde, and D. C. Sullivan. 1996. "Variability in the Interpretation of Screening Mammograms by US Radiologists." *Archives of Internal Medicine* 156(2): 209–213.

Beam, C. M., D. C. Sullivan, and P. M. Layde. 1996. "Effect of Human Variability on Independent Double Reading in Screening Mammography." *Academic Radiology* 3(11): 891–897.

Beaulieu, Anne. 2000. "The Brain at the End of the Rainbow: The Promises of Brain Scans in the Research Field and in the Media." In *Wild Science: Reading Feminism, Medicine, and the Media*, edited by J. Marchessault and K. Sawchuk, 39–52. New York: Routledge.

———. 2002. "Images Are Not the (Only) Truth: Brain Mapping, Visual Knowledge, and Iconoclasm." *Science, Technology, and Human Values* 271:53–86.

Bell, Robert. 2001. "MRI Utilization Mystery." *Decisions in Imaging Economics: The Journal of Imaging Technology Management.* Retrieved March 10, 2005 (http://www.imagingeconomics.com/library).

———. 2004. "Magnetic Resonance in Medicine in 2020." *Decisions in Imaging Economics: The Journal of Imaging Technology Management.* Retrieved March 10, 2005 (http://www.imagingeconomics.com/library).

Bender, Ellen. 2004. "Blaming the Hospitals." *Boston Globe* (September 6): A15.

Berg, Marc, and Annemarie Mol, eds. 1998. *Differences in Medicine: Unraveling Practices, Techniques, and Bodies.* Durham, NC: Duke University Press.

Berger, Arthur. 2003. *Ads, Fads, and Consumer Culture: Advertising's Impact on American Character and Society.* New York: Rowman and Littlefield.

Berger, John. 1973. *Ways of Seeing.* New York: Viking Press.

Bernstein, Barton. 1997. "The Misguided Quest for the Artificial Heart." In *The Sociology of Health and Illness,* 5th ed., edited by Peter Conrad, 352–358. New York: St. Martin's Press.

Bernstein, Douglas, and Peggy Nash. 2001. *Essentials of Psychology.* 2nd ed. Boston: Houghton Mifflin.

Bhargavan, Mythreyi, and Jonathan Sunshine. 2005. "Workload of Radiologists in the United States in 2002–2003 and Trends Since 1991–2." *Radiology* 236(3): 920–939.

Bijker, Wiebe. 1995. *Of Bicycles, Bakelites, and Bulbs: Toward a Theory of Sociotechnical Change.* Cambridge, MA: MIT Press.

Biomedical Market Newsletter. 1998a. "US Industry and Trade Outlook 1998: Global Prospects." *Biomedical Market Newsletter* 8(2): 63.

———. 1998b. "Market Research Studies: Orthopedic Market Leadership Changing from J&J–DePuy Deal." *Biomedical Market Newsletter* 8(11): 23.

———. 2000. "Key Market Analysis, 1999." *Biomedical Market Newsletter* 10(1): 18.

Blewett, Mary. 1988. *Men, Women, and Work: Class, Gender, and Protest in the New England Shoe Industry, 1780–1910.* Chicago: University of Illinois Press.

Blume, Stuart. 1992. *Insight and Industry: On the Dynamics of Technological Change in Medicine.* Cambridge, MA: MIT Press.

Bowman, Lee. 2000. "Studies Test Value of Cancer Screening." *The Chicago Sun Times* (September 20): 5.

Bradsher, Keith. 2002. *High and Mighty: SUVs—the World's Most Dangerous Vehicles and How They Got That Way.* New York: Public Affairs.

Brand, Rachel. 2004. "Souvenir Sonograms: Firms Draw Criticism for Selling Ultrasound Memories to Parents." *Rocky Mountain News* (August 9): B1.

Brass, Larisa. 2005. "New PET Policy Boosts CTI Shares: Reimbursement Plan to Allow Payment for Scans to Detect, Monitor Cancer." *Knoxville News–Sentinel* (February 1): C1.

Brilla, Roland, Stefan Evers, Angela Deutschlander, and Katja Elfriede Wartenberg. 2006. "Are Neurology Residents in the United States Being Taught Defensive Medicine." *Clinical Neurology and Neurosurgery* 108(4): 374–377.

Brockway, J. P., and P. R. Bream. 1992. "Does Memory Loss Occur After MR Imaging?" *Journal of Magnetic Resonance Imaging* 2:721–728.

Brown, Phil, and Edwin Mikkelsen. 1990. *No Safe Place: Toxic Waste, Leukemia, and Community Action.* Berkeley: University of California Press.

Bryson, Norman, ed. 1994. *Visual Culture: Images and Interpretation.* Hanover, NH: University of New England Press for Wesleyan University Press.

Cahan, Vicky, and Doug Dollemore. 2004. "National Institute of Aging, Industry Launch Partnership, $60 Million Alzheimer's Disease NeuroImaging Initiative." *US Department of Health, and Human Services National Institutes of Health Press Release.* Retrieved September 28, 2007 (http://www.nia.nih.gov/NewsAndEvents/PressReleases/PR20041013Neuro.htm).

Canadian Institute for Heath Information [CIHI]. 2005. *Medical Imaging in Canada, 2004.* Ottawa, Ontario: CIHI Publications.

Carey, Timothy, and Joanne Garrett. 1996. "Patterns of Ordering Diagnostic Tests for Patients with Acute Low Back Pain." *Annals of Internal Medicine* 125(10): 807–814.

Carrino, J. A., and F. A. Jolesz. 2005. "MRI-Guided Interventions." *Academic Radiology* 12:1063–1064.

Cartwright, Lisa. 1995. *Screening the Body: Tracing Medicine's Visual Culture.* Minneapolis: University of Minnesota Press.

———. 1998. "A Cultural Anatomy of the Visible Human Project." In *The Visible Woman: Imaging Technologies, Gender, and Science,* edited by Lisa Cartwright, Paula Treichler, and Constance Penley, 21–43. New York: New York University Press.

Cartwright, Lisa, and Brian Goldfarb. 1992. "Radiography, Cinematography and the Decline of the Lens." In *Zone 6: Incorporations,* edited by Jonathan Crary and Sanford Kwinter, 190–201. Cambridge, MA: MIT Press.

Cartwright, Lisa, Paula Treichler, and Constance Penley, eds. 1998. *The Visible Woman: Imaging Technologies, Gender, and Science.* New York: New York University Press.

Casper, Monica. 1998. *The Making of the Unborn Patient: A Social Anatomy of Fetal Surgery.* New Brunswick, NJ: Rutgers University Press.

Cebuhar, Barbara. 2006. Public Affairs Specialist. *Centers for Medicare and Medicaid Services,* personal correspondence.

Center for Devices and Radiological Health (CDRH). 1998. "Guidance for Industry: Guidance for the Submission of Premarket Notifications for Magnetic Resonance Diagnostic Devices." *Food and Drug Administration.* Retrieved September 26, 2007 (http://www.fda.gov/cdrh/ode/mri340.pdf).

Centers for Medicare and Medicaid Services [CMS]. 2006. Medicare Coverage Database. Retrieved June 22, 2006 (http://www.cms.hhs.gov/mcd/results.asp?show=all&t=2006622175417).

Clarke, Adele. 1995. "Modernity, Postmodernity, and Reproductive Processes ca. 1890–1990 or, 'Mommy, Where Do Cyborgs Come From Anyway?'" In *The Cyborg Handbook,* edited by C. H. Gray, H. J. Figueroa-Sarriera, and S. Mentor, 139–155. New York: Routledge.

———. 2004. *Situational Analysis: Grounded Theory after the Postmodern Turn.* Thousand Oaks, CA: Sage.

Clarke, Adele, and Joan Fujimura, eds. 1992. *The Right Tools for the Job.* Princeton, NJ: Princeton University Press.

Clarke, Adele, Janet Shim, Laura Mamo, Jennifer Fosket, and Jennifer Fishman. 2003. "Biomedicalization: Technoscientific Transformations of Health, Illness, and U.S. Biomedicine." *American Sociological Review* 68(2): 161–194.

Collins, Harry. 1974. "The TEA Set: Tacit Knowledge and Scientific Networks." *Science Studies* 4(2): 165–186.

———. 2001. "Tacit Knowledge, Trust and the Q of Sapphire." *Social Studies of Science* 31(1): 71–85.

Collins, Harry, and Martin Kusch. 1998. *The Shape of Actions: What Humans and Machines Can Do.* Cambridge, MA: MIT Press.

Computer Retrieval of Information on Scientific Projects [CRISP]. 2005. "Current and Historical Awards (1972–2005)." Retrieved February 2005 (*http://crisp.cit.nih.gov/*).

Conrad, Peter. 2007. *The Medicalization of Society: On the Transformation of Human Conditions into Treatable Disorders.* Baltimore: John Hopkins University Press.

Conrad, Peter, and Joseph Schneider. 1992 [1980]. *Deviance and Medicalization: From Badness to Sickness.* Philadelphia: Temple University Press.

Cook, Gareth. 2001. "New Brain Map May Highlight Roots of Trouble." *Boston Globe* (May 1): C1, C3.

Copnell, Beverley, Linda Johnston, Denise Harrison, Anita Wilson, Anne Robson, Caroline Mulcahy, Louisa Ramudu, Geraldine McDonnell, and Christine Best. 2004. "Doctors' and Nurses' Perceptions of Interdisciplinary Collaboration in the NICU, and the Impact of a Neonatal Nurse Practitioner Model of Practice." *Journal of Clinical Nursing* 13(1): 105–113.

Corbin, Alain. 1986. *The Foul and the Fragment: Odor and the French Social Imagination.* Cambridge, MA: Harvard University Press.

———. 1998. *Village Bells: Sound and Meaning in the 19th Century French Countryside.* New York: Columbia University Press.

Cornwell, Patricia. 2005. *Predator.* New York: G. P. Putnam's Sons.

Cowan, Ruth Schwartz. 1983. *More Work for Mother: The Ironies of Household Technology from the Open Hearth to the Microwave.* New York: Basic Books.

———. 1987. "The Consumption Junction: A Proposal for Research Strategies in the Sociology of Technology." In *The Social Construction of Technological Systems,* edited by Wiebe Bijker, Thomas Hughes, and Trevor Pinch, 261–280. Cambridge, MA: MIT Press.

Cozzens, Susan, and Edward Woodhouse. 1995. "Science, Government, and the Politics of Knowledge." In *Handbook of Science and Technology Studies,* edited by S. Jasanoff, G. Markle, J. Petersen, and T. Pinch, 533–553. Thousand Oaks, CA: Sage.

Cranberg, Lee, Thomas Glick, and Luke Sato. 2007. "Do the Claims Hold Up? A Study of Medical Negligence Claims against Neurologists." *Journal of Empirical Legal Issues* 4(1): 155–162.

Crary, Jonathan. 1990. *Techniques of the Observer: On Vision and Modernity in the Nineteenth Century.* Cambridge, MA: MIT Press.

———. 1999. *Suspensions of Perception: Attention, Spectacle, and Modern Culture.* Cambridge, MA: MIT Press.

Crooks, Lawrence. 2000. Personal correspondence, September 15.

Cruikshank, Margaret. 2002. *Learning to Be Old: Gender, Culture, and Aging*. New York: Rowan and Littlefield.

Damadian, Raymond. 1971. "Tumor Detection by Nuclear Magnetic Resonance." *Science* 171(3966): 1151–1153.

———. 2000. Personal interview, October 12.

Damadian, Raymond, M. Goldsmith, and L. Minkoff. 1978. "NMR in Cancer: XX. Fonar Scans of Patients with Cancer." *Physiological Chemistry and Physics* 10:285–287.

Dao, James. 1993. "Compromise on Rent Law Is Criticized." *New York Times* (July 5): A23.

Daston, Lorraine, and Peter Galison. 1992. "The Image of Objectivity." *Representations* 40:81–128.

Davies, Karen. 2003. "The Body and Doing Gender: The Relations between Doctors and Nurses in Hospital Work." *Sociology of Health and Illness* 25(7): 720–742.

DeJohn, Paula. 2005. "In Contrast With 1990s, Media Prices Set to Rise." *Hospital Material Management* 30(5): 1–2.

Department of Radiation Sciences [DRS]. 2006. Program in Radiography at Virginia Commonwealth University. Retrieved June 20, 2006 (http://www.sahp .vcu.edu/radsci/radiography.htm).

Diagnostic Imaging Online [DIO]. 2006. "NIH Showers 2006 Grants on Radiology Research," Retrieved November 28, 2006 (http://www.diagnosticimaging .com/showNews.jhtml?articleID=192503724).

Diamond, Timothy. 1992. *Making Gray Gold: Narratives of Nursing Home Care*. Chicago: University of Chicago Press.

Doing, Park. 2003. "Velvet Revolutions: Accounting for Epistemic and Political Change at a Modern Physics Laboratory amid the Second Rise of Biology in Synchrotron Science." Ph.D. diss., Cornell University.

Dowling, Claudia. 1997. "From DaVinci's Drawings to the CAT Scan, Images of the Body Have Fascinated Artists and Doctors." *Life* (February): 48–56.

Duffin, Jacalyn, and Charles Hayter. 2000. "Baring the Sole: The Rise and Fall of the Shoe–Fitting Fluoroscope." *Isis* 91(2): 260–282.

Dumit, Joseph. 1995. "Twenty-first-Century PET: Looking for Mind and Morality through the Eye of Technology." In *Technoscientific Imaginaries: Conversations, Profiles, and Memoirs*, edited by George Marcus, 87–128. Chicago: University of Chicago Press.

———. 1999. "Objective Brains, Prejudicial Images." *Science in Context* 12(1): 173–201.

———. 2000. "When Explanations Rest: 'Good-Enough' Brain Science and the New Socio-Medical Disorders." In *Living and Working with the New Medical Technologies: Intersections of Inquiry*, edited by Margaret Lock, Allan Young, and Alberto Cambrosio, 233–262. New York: Cambridge University Press.

———. 2004. *Picturing Personhood: Brain Scans and Biomedical Identity*. Princeton, NJ: Princeton University Press.

Durkheim, Emile. 1995 [1912]. *The Elementary Forms of Religious Life*. Translated by Karen Fields. New York: The Free Press.

Duster, Troy. 2005. "Race and Reification in Science." *Science* 307(5712): 1050–1051.

Edelstein, W., J. Hutchison, F. Smith, J. Mallard, G. Johnson, and T. Redpath. 1981. "Human Whole-Body NMR Tomographic Imaging: Normal Sections." *British Journal of Radiology* 54(638): 149–151.

Eisner, Marc, Jeff Worsham, and Evan Ringquist. 2000. *Contemporary Regulatory Policy*. Boulder, CO: Lynne RiennerPublishers.

Elmore, Joann, Stephen Taplin, William Barlow, Gary Cutter, Carl D'Orsi, R. Edward Hendrick, Linn Abrham, Jessica Fosse, and Patricia Carney. 2005. "Does Litigation Influence Medical Practice? The Influence of Community Radiologists' Malpractice." *Radiology* 236(1): 37–45.

European Magnetic Resonance Forum [EMRF]. 2005. "Frequently Asked Questions." Retrieved January 2005 (http://www.emrf.org/).

———. 2007. "How Many MR Systems Are There?" Retrieved September 24, 2007 (http://www.emrf.org/New%20Site/FAQs/FAQs%20How%20many%20MRI %20are%20there.htm).

Evans, Robert, Jonathan Lomas, Morris Barer, Roberta Labelle, Catherine Fooks, Gregory Stoddart, Geoffrey Anderson, David Feeny, Amiram Gafni, George Torrance, and William Tholl. 1998. "Controlling Health Expenditures—The Canadian Reality." In *How to Choose? A Comparison of the US and Canadian Healthcare Systems,* edited by Robert Chernomas and Ardeshir Sepehri, 9–22. Amityville, NY: Baywood Publishing Co.

Falkenstein, Jeffrey, ed. 2003. *National Guide to Funding in Health, Eighth Edition.* New York: The Foundation Center.

Fausto-Sterling, Anne. 2004. "Refashioning Race: DNA and the Politics of Health Care." *Differences: A Journal of Feminist Cultural Studies* 15(3): 1–37.

Felner, Julie. 1997. "Dr. Susan Love Cuts through the Hype on Women's Health." *Ms.* (July/August): 37–46.

Ferber, Dan. 2001. "Beyond Polygraphs: Brain Images Tell the Truth." *BioMedNet News and Features.* Retrieved November 6, 2002 (*http://bmn.com/news/story?*).

Fishman, Jennifer. 2004. "Manufacturing Desire: The Commodification of Female Sexual Dysfunction." *Social Studies of Science* 34(2): 187–218.

Fleck, Ludwig. 1979. *Genesis and Development of a Scientific Fact.* Chicago: University of Chicago Press.

Food and Drug Association [FDA]. 2003. "Full-Body CT Scans: What You Need to Know." DHHS Publication No. (FDA) 03–0001. The brochure is available online at http://www.fda.gov/cdrh/ct/ctscansbro.html.

Ford, E., J. Newman, and K. Deosaransing. 2000. "Racial and Ethnic Differences in the Use of Cardiovascular Procedures: Findings from the California Cooperative Cardiovascular Project." *American Journal of Public Health* 90(7): 1128–1134.

Ford, Henry. 1926. *Today and Tomorrow.* New York: Doubleday, Page, and Co.

Foucault, Michel. 1975. *The Birth of the Clinic: An Archeology of Medical Perception.* New York: Vintage Books.

———. 1979. *Discipline and Punish: The Birth of the Prison.* New York: Random House.

———. 1990. *The History of Sexuality,* Vol. 1, *An Introduction.* New York: Vintage Books.

Fox, Renée, and Judith Swazey. 1992. *Spare Parts: Organ Replacement in American Society.* New York: Oxford University Press.

Fuchs, Victor, and James Hahn. 1998. "How Does Canada Do It? A Comparison of Expenditures for Physicians' Services in the United States and Canada." In *How to Choose? A Comparison of the US and Canadian Healthcare Systems*, edited by Robert Chernomas and Ardeshir Sepehri, 23–39. Amityville, NY: Baywood.

Gaeta, Michele, Fabio Minutoli, Emanuele Scribano, Giorgio Ascenti, Sergio Vinci, Daniele Bruschetta, Ludovico Magaudda, and Alfredo Blandino. 2005. "CT and MR Imaging Findings in Athletes with Early Tibial Stress Injuries: Comparison with Bone Scintigraphy Findings and Emphasis on Cortical Abnormalities." *Radiology* 235(2): 553–562.

Garrity-Blake, Barbara. 1994. *The Fish Factory: Work and Meaning for Black and White Fishermen of the American Menhaden Industry*. Knoxville: University of Tennessee Press.

Garza, Cynthia. 2005. "Using Prenatal Ultrasounds as Keepsakes Grows More Popular and Controversial: FDA and Others Question Ethics of the Procedure in Nonmedical Uses." *Houston Chronicle* (August 2): A1.

Gawande, Atul. 2002. *Complications: A Surgeon's Notes on an Imperfect Science*. New York: Metropolitan Books.

Gelb, H., S. Glasgow, A. Sapega, and J. Torg. 1996. "MRI of Knee Disorders: Clinical Value and Cost-Effectiveness in a Sports Medicine Practice." *American Journal of Sports Medicine* 24(1): 99–103.

Gerston, Larry, Cynthia Fraleigh, and Robert Schwab. 1988. *The Deregulated Society*. Pacific Grove, CA: Brooks/Cole.

Glaser, Barney, and Anselm Strauss. 1967. *The Discovery of Grounded Theory: Strategies for Qualitative Research*. Chicago: Aldine.

Glick, Thomas, Lee Cranberg, Robert Hanscom, and Luke Sato. 2005. "Neurologic Patient Safety: An In-Depth Study of Malpractice Claims." *Neurology* 65: 1284–1286.

Golan, Tal. 1998. "The Authority of Shadows: The Legal Embrace of the X-ray." *Historical Reflections* 24(3): 437–458.

Goodwin, Charles. 1994. "Professional Vision." *American Anthropologist* 96(3): 606–633.

———. 1995. "Seeing in Depth." *Social Studies of Science* 25(2): 237–274.

Gordon, Suzanne. 2005. *Nursing Against the Odds: How Health Care Cost Cutting, Media Stereotypes, and Medical Hubris Undermine Nurses and Patient Care*. Ithaca, NY: Cornell University Press.

Gotzsche, P. C., and O. Olsen. 2000. "Is Screening For Breast Cancer Justifiable?" *Lancet* 355(9198): 129–134.

Graham, Sarah. 2005. "Brain Scans Helps Scientists 'Read' Minds." *Scientific American.com*. Retrieved April 26, 2005 (http://www.sciam.com/article.cfm?articleID=000BB5F3-67BE-1269-A7BE83414B7F0000).

Grant, David, and Robin Harris, eds. 1996. *Encyclopedia of Nuclear Magnetic Resonance: Volume One Historical Perspectives*. New York: John Wiley and Sons.

Greider, Katharine. 2003. *The Big Fix: How the Pharmaceutical Industry Rips Off American Consumers*. New York: Public Affairs.

Grey, S. J., G. Price, and A. Mathews. "Reduction of Anxiety During MR Imaging: A Controlled Trial." *Magnetic Resonance Imaging* 18(3): 351–355.

Grosz, Elizabeth. 1994. *Volatile Bodies: Toward a Corporeal Feminism.* Bloomington: Indiana University Press.

Guillemin, Jeanne. 1994. "Experiment and Illusion in Reproductive Medicine." *Human Nature* 5(1): 1–22.

Guillemin, Jeanne, and Lynda Holmstrom. 1999. *Mixed Blessings: Intensive Care for Newborns.* New York: Oxford University Press.

Gusterson, Hugh. 1996. *Nuclear Rites: A Weapons Laboratory at the End of the Cold War.* Berkeley: University of California Press.

Ham, C. L., J. M. Engels, G. T. van de Wiel, and A. Machielsen. 1997. "Peripheral Nerve Stimulation During MRI: Effects of High Gradient Amplitudes and Switching Rates." *Journal of Magnetic Resonance Imaging* 7:933–937.

Haney, Daniel. 2000. "Device Helps Doctors Find Strokes Better." *Chicago Sun-Times* (February 13): 29.

Haraway, Donna. 1988. "Situated Knowledges: The Science Question in Feminism as a Site of Discourse on the Privilege of Partial Perspectives." *Feminist Studies* 14(3): 575–599.

———. 1997. *Modest_Witness@Second_Millenium.FemaleMan©_Meets_Oncomouse™.* New York: Routledge.

———. 2003. *The Companions Species Manifesto: Dogs, People, and Significant Otherness.* Chicago: Prickly Paradigm Press.

Harris, Richard. 2006. Director of Research. American Society of Radiologic Technologists. Personal correspondence.

Harris, Scott. 2006. "Battle Lines Drawn over Specialty Hospitals." *Association of American Medical Colleges Reporter.* Retrieved July 13, 2006 (http://www.aamc.org/newsroom/reporter/may06/specialty.htm).

Hartouni, Valerie. 1997. *Cultural Conceptions: On Reproductive Technologies and the Remaking of Life.* Minneapolis: University of Minnesota Press.

Haydel, M, C. Preston, T. Mills, S. Luber, E. Blaudeau, and P. DeBlieux. 2000. "Indications for Computed Tomography in Patients with Minor Head Injury." *New England Journal of Medicine* 343(2): 138–140.

Hensley, Scott. 1997. "MRI Renaissance: After Being Given Up for Dead a Few Years Ago, Magnetic Resonance Imaging Is Undergoing a Startling Rebirth." *Modern Healthcare* (December 1): 1, 56.

Hilzenrath, David. 1994. "Big N.Y. Health Insurer Weighs Curbs on Policy Coverage, Choice of Doctors." *Washington Post* (November 15): A9.

Himmelberg, Robert, ed. 1994. *Regulatory Issues Since 1964: The Rise of the Deregulation Movement.* New York: Garland.

Hoffman, Jerome, William Mower, Allan Wolfson, Knox Todd, and Michael Tucker. 2000. "Validity of a Set of Clinical Criteria to Rule Out Injury to the Cervical Spine in Patients with Blunt Trauma." *New England Journal of Medicine* 343(2): 94–99.

Hollis, Donald. 1987. *Abusing Cancer Science: The Truth about NMR and Cancer.* Washington, DC: Strawberry Fields Press.

Honey, Martha. 1995. "Pesticides: Nowhere To Hide." *Ms.* (July/August): 16–24.

Horstein, Shelley, and Florence Jacobowitz, eds. 2002. *Image and Remembrance: Representation and the Holocaust.* Bloomington: Indiana University Press.

Hotz, Robert Lee. 2001. "Byte by Byte: A Map of the Brain." *Los Angeles Times* (July 2): A12.

Hoult, D. 1979. "Rotating Frame Zeugmatography." *Journal of Magnetic Resonance* 33(1): 183.

Huget, Jennifer. 2003. "ADHD Made Visible." *Washington Post* (December 9): HE1.

Information Means Value [IMV]. 2003. "Latest IMV Study Shows Continued Strength in MRI Market as Product Portfolio Broadens." Retrieved October 15, 2005 (http://www.imvlimited.com/mid/pdf/News/1003/MRI%200203–Release–Oct%202003%20(1).pdf).

———. 2005. "Non-hospital Sites Perform Over 40% of All Procedures." Retrieved October 15, 2005 (http://www.imvlimited.com/mid/mri_census.html).

———. 2007. "Latest IMV Market Report Shows Continued High Demand for High Field MRI Systems." Retrieved September 21, 2007 (http://www.invlimited.com/index.aspx?sec=mri&sub=def).

Ingraham, Chrys. 1994. "The Heterosexual Imaginary: Feminist Sociology and Theories of Gender." *Sociological Theory* 12(2): 203–219.

Institute of Medicine [IOM]. 2002. *Unequal Treatment: Confronting Racial and Ethnic Disparities in Health Care.* Washington, DC: National Academy Press.

International Society for Magnetic Resonance in Medicine [ISMRM]. 2006. "ISMRM Questions and Answers." Retrieved June 23, 2006 (http://www.ismrm.org/ISMRMFAQ.htm#2).

Jacobson, P. D., and C. J. Rosenquist. 1996. "The Use of Low-osmolar Contrast Agents: Technological Change and Defensive Medicine," *Journal of Health, Politics, and Law* 21:243–266.

Jarvik, Jeffrey, William Hollingworth, Brook Martin, Scott Emerson, Darryl T. Gray, Steven Overman, David Robinson, Thomas Staiger, Frank Wessbecher, Sean D. Sullivan, William Kreuter, and Richard A. Deyo. 2003. "Rapid Magnetic Resonance Imaging Versus Radiographs for Patients with Low Back Pain." *JAMA* 289(21): 2810–2818.

Jasanoff, Sheila. 1995. *Science at the Bar: Law, Science, and Technology in America.* Cambridge, MA: Harvard University Press.

———. 2006. "Ordering Knowledge, Ordering Society." In *States of Knowledge: The Co-Production of Science and Social Order,* edited by Sheila Jasanoff, 13–45. London: Routledge.

Jay, Martin. 1994. *Downcast Eyes: The Denigration of Vision in Twentieth Century French Thought.* Berkeley: University of California Press.

Jenkins, Reese. 1975. *Images and Enterprise: Technology and the American Photographic Industry, 1839–1925.* Baltimore: Johns Hopkins University Press.

Johnson, Carolyn. 2004. "High-tech Images Open Window into the Skull." *Boston Globe* (September 28): C4.

Joyce, Kelly. 2005. "Appealing Images: Magnetic Resonance Imaging and the Production of Authoritative Knowledge." *Social Studies of Science* 35(3): 437–462.

Kachalia, Allen, Niteesh Choudhry, and David Studdert. 2005. "Physician Responses to the Malpractice Crisis: From Defense to Offense." *Journal of Law, Medicine, and Ethics* 33(3): 416–428.

Kahn, Jennifer. 2001. "Let's Make Your Brain Interactive." *Wired*. Retrieved June 15, 2002 (http://www.loni.ucla.edu/media/News/W_08092001.html).

Kahn, Jonathan. 2005. "Misreading Race and Genomics after BiDil." *Nature Genetics* 37(7): 655–656.

Kaiser, C.P. 2000. "RSNA Continues Disney Partnership and Seeks Additional Sponsors." *Diagnostic Imaging* (November 9): 1–2.

Kanal, Emanuel. 2000. "MRI Safety." Retrieved June 4, 2000 (http://radserv.arad.upmc.edu/MRI_Safety).

Kanal, Emanuel, J. Gillen, J. Evans, D. Savitz, and F. Shellock. 1993. "Survey of Reproductive Health among Female MR Workers." *Radiology* 187:395–399.

Kent, Ann. 1987. "Technology Transfer 2: Progress in Medical Scanners." *Financial Times* (November 10): 16.

Kerber, Ross. 2005. "Drug Makers Adding X-rays, MRIs to Arsenal: Imaging May Help Predict Pharmaceuticals' Effects." *Boston Globe* (January 3): C1, C3.

Kevles, Bettyann. 1997. *Naked to the Bone: Medical Imaging in the Twentieth Century*. New Brunswick, NJ: Rutgers University Press.

Kevles, Daniel. 1987. *The Physicists: The History of a Scientific Community in Modern America*. Cambridge, MA: Harvard University Press.

Kirby, David. 2001. "Patients Embrace New Generation of Imaging Machines." *New York Times* (May 8): D7.

Kleinfield, Sonny. 1985. *A Machine Called Indomitable: The Remarkable Story of a Scientist's Inspiration, Invention, and Medical Breakthrough*. New York: Times Books.

Klingman, D., A. R. Localio, and J. Sugarman. 1996. "Measuring Defensive Medicine Using Clinical Scenario Surveys." *Journal of Health Politics, Policy and Law* 21:185–217.

Kowalczyk, Liz. 2002. "Rush for Medical Scans Raises Concerns on Costs." Excite Media Group. Retrieved March 2005 (http://www.excitepr.com/03b_nia092804.html/).

Krasner, Jeffrey. 2004. "MRI Machines Adapt to Newest Patients: Pets." *Boston Globe* (September 7): F1.

Kroll-Smith, Stephen, Phil Brown, and Valerie Gunter, eds. 2000. *Illness and the Environment: A Reader in Contested Medicine*. New York: New York University Press.

Kroll-Smith, Stephen, and Hugh Floyd. 1997. *Bodies in Protest: Environmental Illness and the Struggle over Medical Knowledge*. New York: New York University Press.

Kumar, A., D. Welti, and R. Ernst. 1975. "NMR-Fourier Zeugmatography." *Journal of Magnetic Resonance* 18:69–83.

Lama, Dalai. 2005. *The Universe in a Single Atom: The Convergence of Science and Spirituality*. New York: Morgan Road Books.

Laming, D., and R. Warren. 2000. "Improving the Detection of Cancer in the Screening of Mammograms." *Journal of Medical Screening* 7(1): 24–30.

Latour, Bruno. 1987. *Science in Action: How to Follow Scientists and Engineers through Society*. Cambridge, MA: Harvard University Press.

———. 1993 [1988]. *The Pasteurization of France*. Cambridge, MA: Harvard University Press.

Latour, Bruno, and Steve Woolgar. 1986 [1979]. *Laboratory Life: The Construction of Scientific Facts*. Princeton, NJ: Princeton University Press.

Lauterbur, Paul. 1973. "Image Formation by Induced Local Interactions: Examples Employing Nuclear Magnetic Resonance." *Nature* 242(March 16): 190–191.

———. 1986. "Cancer Detection by Nuclear Magnetic Resonance Zeugmatographic Imaging." *Cancer* 57:1899–1904.

———. 1996. "One Path of Many—How MRI Actually Began." In *Encyclopedia of Nuclear Magnetic Resonance: Volume One Historical Perspective,* edited by D. Grant and R. Harris, 445–449. New York: John Wiley and Sons.

———. 2000. Personal interview, September 22.

Lauterbur, Paul, David Kramer, William House, and C. Chen. 1975. "Zeugmatographic High Resolution Nuclear Magnetic Resonance Spectroscopy: Images of Chemical Homogeneity within Macroscopic Objects." *Journal of American Chemical Society* 97:6866–6868.

Lessig, Lawrence. 2005. *Free Culture: The Nature and Future of Creativity.* New York: Penguin.

Levitt, Seymour. 1999. "President's Letter." *1999 Scientific Program: Radiological Society of North America* 213:1.

Lewis, Carol. 2001. "Full-Body CT Scans: What You Need to Know." *FDA Consumer Magazine* 35(6): 33.

Library of Congress. 2000. "Project on the Decade of the Brain: Activities." Retrieved June 29, 2006 (http//www.loc.gov/brain/activity.html).

Lillie-Blanton, Marsha, Osula Rushing, and Sonia Ruiz. 2002. *Racial/Ethnic Differences in Cardiac Care: The Weight of the Evidence.* Menlo Park, CA: Henry J. Kaiser Family Foundation Publication no. 6041.

Lim, Michelle. 2002. "Fetal Photos and Body Scans in Parking Lots: The Implications of Bypassing Physicians in the Medical Marketplace." American Medical Association. Retrieved October 2005 (http://www.ama–assn.org/ama/pub/category/9154.html/).

Lim, Tiong Keng, LeahBurden, Rajesh Janardhanan, Chai Ping, James Moon, Dudley Pennell, and Roxy Senior. 2005. "Improved Accuracy of Low-Power Contrast Echocardiography for the Assessment of Left Ventricular Remodeling Compared with Unenhanced Harmonic Echocardiography after Acute Myocardial Infarction: Comparison with Cardiovascular Magnetic Resonance Imaging." *Journal of the American Society of Echocardiography* 18(11): 1203–7.

Linton, Owen. 1997. *The American College of Radiology: The First 75 Years.* Reston, VA: American College of Radiology.

Liu, Stephen, Mark Henry, Stephen Nuccion, Mathew Shapiro, and Fred Dorey. 1996. "Diagnosis of Glenoid Labral Tears: A Comparison Between MRI and Clinical Examinations." *American Journal of Sports Medicine* 24(2): 149–154.

Lock, Margaret. 2002. *Twice Dead: Organ Transplants and the Reinvention of Death.* Berkeley: University of California Press.

Loe, Meika. 2004. *The Rise of Viagra: How the Little Blue Pill Changed Sex in America.* New York: New York University Press.

Lu, Y., and R. Arenson. 2006. "The Academic Radiologist's Clinical Productivity: An Update." *Academic Radiology* 12(9): 1211–1223.

Lundberg, George. 2000. *Severed Trust: Why American Medicine Hasn't Been Fixed.* New York: Basic Books.

Lynch, Michael. 1985a. *Art and Artifact in Laboratory Science: A Study of Shop Work and Shop Talk in a Research Laboratory*. Boston: Routledge and Kegan Paul.

——. 1985b. "Discipline and the Material Form of Images: An Analysis of Scientific Visibility." *Social Studies of Science* 15(1): 37–66.

Lynch, Michael, and Steve Woolgar, eds. 1990. *Representation in Scientific Practice*. Cambridge, MA: MIT Press.

MacKenzie, Donald, and Judy Wajcman, eds. 1985. *The Social Shaping of Technology: How the Refrigerator Got Its Hum*. Philadelphia: Open University Press.

Mallard, John. 1993. "A Brief Personal Account of the Aberdeen Story—with Particular Reference to SPECT and MRI." *Journal of Medical Engineering and Technology* 17(5): 176–179.

——. 2000. Personal interview, September 23.

Mallard, J., J. Hutchison, W. Edelstein, R. Ling, and M. Foster. 1979. "Imaging by Nuclear Magnetic Resonance and Its Bio-medical Implications." *Journal of Biomedical Engineering* 1 (July): 153–160.

Mamo, Laura. 2007. *Queering Reproduction: Achieving Pregnancy in the Age of Technoscience*. Durham, NC: Duke University Press.

Mansfield, Peter, and Grannell, Paul. 1973. *Journal of Physics C* 6: L422.

Mansfield, P., and A. Maudsley. 1977. "Medical Imaging by NMR." *British Journal of Radiology* 50(591): 188–194.

Marks, Harry. 1997. *The Progress of Experiment: Science and Therapeutic Reform in the United States, 1990–1990*. New York: Cambridge University Press.

Martin, Brian, and Evelleen Richards. 1995. "Scientific Knowledge, Controversy, and Public Decision Making." In *Handbook of Science and Technology Studies*, edited by S. Jasanoff, G. Markle, J. Petersen, and T. Pinch, 506–526. Thousand Oaks, CA: Sage.

Martin, Emily. 1987. *The Woman in the Body: A Cultural Analysis of Reproduction*. Boston: Beacon Press.

——. 1995. *Flexible Bodies: The Role of Immunity in American Culture from the Days of Polio to the Age of Aids*. Boston: Beacon Press.

Matin, A., D. Bates, A. Sussman, P. Ros, R. Hanson, and R. Khorasani. 2006. "Inpatient Radiology Utilization: Trends over the Past Decade." *American Journal of Roentgenology* 186(1): 7–11.

Mattson, J., and M. Simon, M. 1996. *The Pioneers of NMR and Magnetic Resonance in Medicine: The Story of MRI*. New York: Dean Books.

McAllister, Matthew. 1995. *The Commercialization of American Culture: New Advertising, Control, and Democracy*. Thousand Oaks, CA: Sage.

McCarthy, Terry. 2005. "Getting Inside Your Head: As 'Neuro' Goes Mainstream, Big Business Hopes to Decode the Brain's Secrets." *Time* 166(17): 94–97.

McCullough, Michael, Tadeusz Jezierski, Michael Broffman, Alan Hubbard, Kirk Turner, and Teresa Janecki. 2006. "Diagnostic Accuracy of Canine Scent Detection in Early- and Late-Stage Lung and Breast Cancers." *Integrative Cancer Therapies* 5(1): 30–39.

McGibbon, K. A. 1998. "Evidence Based Practice." *Bulletin of the Medical Library Association* 86(3): 396–401.

McKeown, Thomas, R. G. Brown, and R. G. Record. 1972. "An Interpretation of the Modern Rise of Population in Europe." *Population Studies* 26(3): 345–382.

McKeown, Thomas, R. G. Record, and R. D. Turner. 1975. "An Interpretation of the Decline of Mortality in England and Wales During the Twentieth Century." *Population Studies* 29: 391–422.

McKinlay, John, and Sonja McKinlay. 1997. "Medical Measures and the Decline of Mortality." In *The Sociology of Health and Illness*, 5th ed., edited by Peter Conrad, 10–23. New York: St. Martin's Press.

Medical and Healthcare Marketplace Guide. 1998a. "Contrast Agents—Market Evolution: Part I." *A Series of Reports on Contrast Agents*. London, UK: Datamonitor Group.

———. 1998b. "Contrast Agents—Background: Part II." *A Series of Reports on Contrast Agents*. London, UK: Datamonitor Group.

Melendez, J. C., and E. McCrank. 1993. "Anxiety-related Reactions Associated with Magnetic Resonance Imaging Examinations." *JAMA* 270(6): 745–747.

Merrill, Richard. 1994. "Regulation of Drugs and Devices: An Evolution." *Health Affairs* 13(3): 47–69.

———. 1999. "Modernizing the FDA: An Incremental Revolution." *Health Affairs* 18(2): 96–111.

Miller, A. B., T. To, C. J. Baines, and C. Wall. 2002. "The Canadian National Breast Screening Study-1: Breast Cancer Mortality After 11 to 16 Years of Follow-Up." *Annals of Internal Medicine* 137: 305–312.

Mirzoeff, Nicholas, ed. 1998. *Visual Culture Reader*. New York: Routledge.

Mitchell, William J. 1994. *Picture Theory: Essays on Verbal and Visual Representation*. Chicago: University of Chicago Press.

Mol, Annemarie. 2002. *The Body Multiple: Ontology in Medical Practice*. Durham, NC: Duke University Press.

Moore, Lisa Jean. 1997. " 'It's Like You Use Pots and Pans to Cook. It's the Tool': The Technologies of Safer Sex." *Science, Technology, and Human Values* 22(4): 434–471.

Mudambi, Ram, ed. 2003. *Privatization and Globalization: The Changing Role of the State in Business*. Northampton, MA: Edward Elgar Press.

Munsey, Robert. 1995. "Trends and Events in FDA Regulation of Medical Devices over the Last Fifty Years." *Food and Drug Law Journal* 50: 163–177.

Murphy, K. J., and J. A. Brumberg. 1997. "Adult Claustrophobia, Anxiety, and Sedation in MRI." *Magnetic Resonance Imaging* 15(1): 51–54.

Murphy, Michelle. 2006. *Sick Building Syndrome and the Problem of Uncertainty*. Durham, NC: Duke University Press.

Myers, David. 2003. *Psychology*. 7th ed. New York: Worth.

National Electrical Manufacturers Association [NEMA]. 1999. "Domestic Shipments of Select Product Groups within the Scope of NEMA's Diagnostic Imaging and Therapy Systems Division." Retrieved June 10, 2001 (http://www.nema.org/economics/factfig99/domship/div9html).

National Institute of Aging [NIA]. 2006. "Alzheimer's Disease Neuroimaging Study Launched Nationwide by the National Institutes of Health." Retrieved October 25, 2006 (http://www.nia.nih.gov/Alzheimers/ResearchInformation/NewsReleases/PR20060209.htm).

National Institute of Biomedical Imaging and Bioengineering [NIBIB]. 2006. "NIBIB Grantee Awarded Gold Medal by International Society for Magnetic Resonance in Medicine." May 23 News Release. Retrieved June 24, 2006 (http://www.nibib.nih.gov/NewsEvents/Releases#May).

National Institute of Mental Health [NIMH]. 2002. "Neuroinformatics: The Human Brain Project Home." Retrieved March 20, 2003 (http://www.nimh.nih.gov/neuroinformatics/index.cfm).

Navarro, Vicente. 1993. *Dangerous to Your Health: Capitalism in Health Care.* New York: Monthly Review Press.

Neve, Clare. 2004. "What's Up, Dog? Another Top Diagnosis." *Daily Telegraph* (November 10): 18.

Nordenberg, Tamar. 1999. "The Picture of Health: It's What's Inside That Counts with X-rays, Other Imaging Methods." *FDA Consumer* 33(1): 8–13.

Novello, Antonia. 2002. "DOH Medicaid Update: Magnetic Resonance Imaging—Physician and Clinic Billing." Office of Medicaid Management. Retrieved June 27, 2006 (http://www.health .state.ny.us/health_care/medicaid/program/update/2002/may2002.htm#mri).

Oakley, Ann. 1984. *The Captured Womb: A History of the Medical Care of Pregnant Women.* New York: Blackwell.

Office of Technology Assessment [OTA]. (1984) *Health Technology Case Study 27: Nuclear Magnetic Resonance Imaging Technology: A Clinical, Industrial, and Policy Analysis.* Washington, DC: U.S. Government Printing Office, OTA-HCS-27.

Ogle, Peter. 2001. "MRI, CT, and PET Present Formidable Imaging Triumvirate." *Diagnostic Imaging* 23(5): 7.

Olden, Kenneth. 1999. *NIEHS Report on Health Effects from Exposure to Power-Line Frequency Electric and Magnetic Fields.* Rockville, MD: NIH Publication No. 99–4493.

Olney, Buster. 2002. "Pro Football: Giants Notebook; For Hilliard, Serenity Vanishes in a Second." *New York Times* (October 30): D2.

Oudshoorn, Nelly. 1994. *Beyond the Natural Body: An Archeology of Sex Hormones.* New York: Routledge.

———. 2003. *The Male Pill: A Biography of a Technology in the Making.* Durham, NC: Duke University Press.

Oudshoorn, Nelly, and Trevor Pinch, ed. 2005. *How Users Matter: The Co-Construction of Users and Technology.* Cambridge, MA: MIT Press.

Ouwendijk, Rody, Marianne de Vries, Peter M. T. Pattynama, Marc R. H. M. van Sambeek, Michiel W. de Haan, Teho Stijnen, Jos M. A. van Engelshoven, and M. G. Myriam Hunink. 2005. "Imaging Peripheral Arterial Disease: A Randomized Controlled Trial Comparing Contrast-enhanced MR Angiography and Multi-Detector Row CT Angiography." *Radiology* 235(9): 1094–1103.

Oxford English Dictionary (OED). 1989. Oxford, UK: Clarendon Press.

Palosky, Craig. 1995. "Doctor's Orders: When Corporate Rule-Makers Restrict Treatment Options, a Patient May Suffer From Bad Medical Decisions for Which Neither the Doctor nor the Insurer Accepts Total Responsibility." *Tampa Tribune* (September 3): 1.

Panati, Charles. 1991. *Panati's Parade of Fads, Follies, and Manias: The Origins of Our Cherished Obsessions.* New York: HarperCollins.

Parlette, Alicia. "Alice's Story: Cancer, Despair, Hope, Faith." *San Francisco Chronicle* (September 30): E1.

Pasveer, Bernike. 1989. "Knowledge of Shadows: The Introduction of X-ray Images in Medicine." *Sociology of Health and Illness* 11(4): 360–381.

Paulsen, Monte. 1993. "The Politics of Cancer: Why the Medical Establishment Blames Victims Instead of Carcinogens." *Utne Reader* (November/December): 81–89.

Payer, Lynn. 1996 [1988]. *Medicine and Culture: Varieties of Treatment in the United States, England, West Germany, and France.* New York: Henry Holt.

Pierce, Alan. 2006. "2004–2005 Survey of New York Law: Insurance Law." *Syracuse Law Review* 56(4): 881–930.

Pinch, Trevor, and Wiebe Bijker. 1984. "The Social Construction of Facts and Artifacts: Or How the Sociology of Science and the Sociology of Technology Might Benefit Each Other." *Social Studies of Science* 13: 399–431.

Plotnick, Rod. 2001. *Introduction to Psychology (with Infotrac).* Belmont, CA: Wadsworth.

Polanyi, Karl. 2001 [1944]. *The Great Transformation: The Political and Economic Origins of Our Time.* Boston: Beacon Press.

Poling, Travis. 2004. "The Big Buzz Is Magnets; Once Rare, MRI Machines Have Become Common and Profitable." *San Antonio Express–News* (June 19): D1.

Porter, Theodore. 1995. *Trust in Numbers: The Pursuit of Objectivity in Science and Public Life.* Princeton, NJ: Princeton University Press.

Prasad, Amit. 2005a. "Scientific Culture in the 'Other' Theater of 'Modern Science': An Analysis of the Culture of Magnetic Resonance Imaging Research in India." *Social Studies of Science* 35(3): 463–490.

———. 2005e. "Making Images/Making Bodies: Visibilizing and Disciplining through Magnetic Resonance Imaging." *Science, Technology and Human Values* 30(2): 291–316.

Proto, Anthony. 2004. "Radiology 2004—New Directions." *Radiology* 230(1): 3–5.

Quirk, M. E., A. J. Letendre, R. A. Ciottone, and J. F. Lingley. 1989. "Anxiety in Patients Undergoing MR Imaging." *Radiology* 170(2): 463–466.

Radiological Society of North America [RSNA]. 2000. "RSNA News—September 2000." Retrieved April 13, 2001 (http://wwww.rsna.org/publications/rsnanews/sept00/pcc.html).

———. 2003. "Salaries Rise for Radiologists in 2002." Retrieved May 15, 2004 (http://www.rsna.org/publications/rsnanews/oct03/salaries-1.htm).

———. 2005a. "History of the Radiological Society of North America." Retrieved October 12, 2005 (http://www.rsna.org/about/history/articles.html).

———. 2005b. "Salaries Flat for Interventional Diagnostic Radiologists." *RSNA News* 15 (10): 8–9. (http://www.rsna.org/publications/rsnanews/oct03/salaries-1.htm).

———. 2005c. "Meeting Facts." Retrieved December 5, 2006 (http://www.rsna.org/Media/rsna/upload/Meeting_Facts_2005.pdf).

Radford, Tim. 2001. "Brain Images Show Appeal Lies in the Blink of an Eye." *The Guardian* (October 11): 15.

Reiser, Stanley Joel. 1978. *Medicine and the Reign of Technology.* New York: Cambridge University Press.

Relman, Arnold. 1997a. "The Health Care Industry: Where Is It Taking Us?" In *The Sociology of Health and Illness*, 5th ed., edited by Peter Conrad, 240–246. New York: St. Martin's Press.

———. 1997b. "The Market for Health Care: Where Is the Patient?" *Clinical Chemistry* 43(12): 2225–2229.

Ritter, Jim. 2000. "Scanner Can Find Cancer, But Not All Doctors Sold." *Chicago-Sun Times* (October 18): 28.

Rose N. E., and S. M. Gold. 1996. "A Comparison of Accuracy Between Clinical Examination and Magnetic Resonance Imaging in the Diagnosis of Meniscal and Anterior Cruciate Ligament Tears." *Arthroscopy* 12(4): 398–405.

Rosenstein, A. H. 2002. "Nurse-Physician Relationships: Impact on Nurse Satisfaction and Retention." *American Journal of Nursing* 102(6): 26–33.

Ross, Elizabeth. 1993. "Landlords in Mass. Fight Rent Control." *Christian Science Monitor* (November 29): 1.

Roth, Julius. 1997. "Some Contingencies of the Moral Evaluation and Control of Clientele: The Case of the Hospital Emergency Service." In *The Sociology of Health and Illness*, 5th ed., edited by Peter Conrad, 247–259. New York: St. Martin's Press.

Sackett, David, W., M. C. Rosenberg, J. A. Gray, B. R. Haynes, and W. S. Richardson. 1996. "Evidence Based Medicine: What It Is and What It Isn't." *British Journal of Medicine* 312(7023): 71–72.

Sackett, David, S. E. Straus, W. S. Richardson, W. Rosenbers, and B. R. Haynes. 2000. *Evidence-Based Medicine: How to Practice and Teach EBM*. New York: Churchill Livingstone.

Sanjiv, Kumra, and Emily Thaden. 2004. "Examining Brain Connectivity in ADHD." *Psychiatric Times* (January): 40–44.

Schenck, John. 2000. "Safety of Strong, Static Magnetic Fields." *Journal of Magnetic Resonance Imaging* 12(1): 2–19.

Schiebinger, Londa. 1993. *Nature's Body: Gender in the Making of Modern Science*. Boston: Beacon Press.

Schild, Hans. 1999. *MRI Made Easy, Well Almost*. New Jersey: Berlex Laboratories.

Schneider, David. 1997. "Raymond V. Damadian: Scanning the Horizon." *Scientific American* 276(6): 32.

Schlosser, Eric. 2002. *Fast Food Nation: What the All American Meal Is Doing to the World*. Gardners Books.

Schor, Juliet. 2004. *Born to Buy: The Commercialized Child and the New Consumer Culture*. New York: Scribner Books.

Schramm, Peter, Peter Schellinger, Ernst Klotz, Kai Kallenberg, Jochen Fiebach, Sonja Külkens, Sabine Heiland, Michael Knauth, and Klaus Sartor. 2004. "Comparison of Perfusion Computer Tomography and Computed Tomography Angiography Source Images with Perfusion-Weighted Imaging and Diffusion-Weighted Imaging in Patients with Acute Stroke of Less Than 6 Hours' Duration." *Stroke* 35(7): 1652–8.

Schulman, K. A., J. A. Berlin, W. Harless, J. F. Kerner, S. Sistrunk, B. J. Gersh, R. Dube, C. K. Taleghani, J. E. Burke, S. Williams, J. Eisenberg, J. J. Escarce, and W. Ayers. 1999. "The Effect of Race and Sex on Physicians' Recommendations for Cardiac Catheterization." *New England Journal of Medicine* 340:618–626.

Segal, David. 1995. "Rockville Firm Makes an Open, Not Shut, Case for MRI." *Washington Post* (December 18): F9.

Shapin, Steven. 1995. *A Social History of Truth: Civility and Science in Seventeenth Century England*. Chicago: University of Chicago Press.

Shapin, Steven, and Simon Schaffer. 1985. *Leviathan and the Air-Pump: Hobbes, Boyle, and the Experimental Life*. Princeton, NJ: Princeton University Press.

Shellock, Frank. 2001. *Guide To MR Procedures and Metallic Objects: Update 2001, Seventh Edition*. Philadelphia: Lippincott, Williams and Wilkins Healthcare.

———. 2001. *Magnetic Resonance Procedures: Health Effects and Safety*. Boca Raton, FL: CRC Press, LLC.

Shellock, Frank, and Howard Bierman. 1989. "The Safety of MRI." *JAMA* 261(23): 3412.

Shellock, Frank, and Emanuel Kanal. 1994. *Magnetic Resonance: Bioeffects, Safety, and Patient Management*. New York: Raven Press.

Shiels, Maggie. 2001. "3D Brain Mappers Scan Thousands." BBC News Online. Retrieved June 26, 2002 (http://www.loni.ucla.edu/media/News/BBC_12062001.htm).

Sismondo, Sergio. 2004. "Pharmaceutical Maneuvers." *Social Studies of Science* 34(2): 149–159.

Skler, K., K. Penn-Jones, M. Cataldo, R. Conner, and E. Zerhouni. 1991. "Music Enhances Patient Comfort during MRI." *American Journal of Radiology* 156:403.

Sontag, Susan. 1990. *On Photography*. New York: Anchor Books.

Squier, Susan. 2004. *Liminal Lives: Imagining the Human at the Frontiers of Biomedicine*. Durham, NC: Duke University Press.

Stabile, Carol. 1993. "Shooting the Mother: Fetal Photography and the Politics of Disappearance." *Camera Obscura* 28(Winter): 179–205.

Stacey, Jackie. 1997. *Teratologies: A Cultural Study of Cancer*. New York: Routledge.

Stafford, Barbara. 1991. *Body Criticism: Imaging the Unseen in Enlightenment Art and Medicine*. Cambridge, MA: MIT Press.

Starr, Paul. 1982. *The Social Transformation of American Medicine*. New York: Basic Books.

———. 1995. "What Happened to Health Care Reform?" *The American Prospect* 20 (Winter): 20–31.

Strauss, Anselm. 1993. *The Permutation of Action*. New York: Aldine de Gruyter.

Strunsky, Steve. 2002. "Center Offers Pets Their Own Place for an MRI, CT Scan." *Associated Press State and Local Wire* (November 11).

Studdert, David, Michelle Mello, William Sage, Catherine DesRoches, Jordon Peugh, Kinga Zapert, and Troyen Brennan. 2005. "Defensive Medicine among High-Risk Specialist Physicians in a Volatile Malpractice Environment." *JAMA* 293(21): 2609–2617.

Sturken, Marita, and Lisa Cartwright. 2001. *Practices of Looking: An Introduction to Visual Culture*. Chicago: University of Chicago Press.

Sullivan, Jean. 2000. "MassHealth Diagnostic and Surgical Bulletin 5." Massachusetts Health and Human Services. Retrieved June 27, 2006 (http://www.mass.gov/Eeohhs2/docs/masshealth/bull_2000/dsf-5.pdf).

Sward, Keith. 1948. *The Legend of Henry Ford*. New York: Rinehart.

Thackray, Arnold, ed. 1998. *Private Science: Biotechnology and the Rise of Molecular Sciences.* Philadelphia: University of Pennsylvania Press.

Thirteen/WNET and BBC-TV. 1993. *Medicine at the Crossroads: Random Cuts.* Produced by Stefan Moore and Martin Freeth. Alexandria, VA: Distributed by PBS Videos.

Thornbury, J. R. 1994. "Why Should Radiologists Be Interested in Technology Assessment and Outcomes Research?" *American Journal of Roentgenology* 163(5): 1027–1030.

Thorpe, D., R. G. Owens, G. Whitehouse, and M. E. Dewey. 1990. "Subjective Experiences of Magnetic Resonance Imaging." *Clinical Radiology* 41(4): 276–278.

Timmermans, Stefan. 1999. *Sudden Death and the Myth of CPR.* Philadelphia: Temple University Press.

Timmermans, Stefan, and Marc Berg. 2003. *The Gold Standard: The Challenge of Evidence-Based Medicine and Standardization in Health Care.* Philadelphia: Temple University Press.

Timmermans, Stefan, and Valerie Leiter. 2000. "The Redemption of Thalidomide: Standardizing the Risk of Birth Defects." *Social Studies of Science* 30(1): 41–71.

Todd, Alexandra Dundas. 1989. *Intimate Adversaries: Cultural Conflicts between Doctors and Women Patients.* Philadelphia: University of Pennsylvania Press.

——. 1994. *Double Vision: An East–West Collaboration for Coping with Cancer.* Hanover, NH: University of New England Press for Wesleyan University Press.

Traweek, Sharon. 1992. *Beamtimes and Lifetimes: The World of High–Energy Physicists.* Cambridge, MA: Harvard University Press.

Tsushima, Yoshito, and Keigo Endo. 2005. "MR Imaging in the Evaluation of Chronic or Recurrent Headache." *Radiology* 235(2): 575–579.

Turnbull, Nancy. 1996. "Managed Care: For People or Profit?" *Sojourner: The Women's Forum* (March): 15–16.

Tuschl, H., G. Neubauer, G. Schmid, E. Weber, and N. Winker. 2000. "Occupational Exposure to Static, ELF, VF, and VLF Magnetic Fields and Immune Parameters." *International Journal of Occupational Medicine and Environmental Health* 13(1): 39–50.

van Dijck, José. 2005. *The Transparent Body: A Cultural Analysis of Medical Imaging.* Seattle: University of Washington Press.

Vidmar, Neil, Kara MacKillop, and Paul Lee. 2006. "Million Dollar Medical Malpractice Cases in Florida: Post-Verdict and Pre-Suit Settlements." *Vanderbilt Law Review* 59(4): 1343–1382.

Volunteer Trustees Foundation. 2006. *The Sale and Conversion of Not–For–Profit Hospitals: A State-by-State Analysis of New Legislation.* Washington, DC: Volunteer Trustees Foundation.

Wahlberg, David. 2004. "Advertisers Probe Brains, Raise Fears." *Atlanta Journal–Constitution* (February 1): 1Q.

Waitzkin, Howard. 1997. "A Marxian Interpretation of the Growth and Development of Coronary Care Technology." In *The Sociology of Health and Illness,* 5th ed., edited by Peter Conrad, 247–259. New York: St. Martin's Press.

Waldby, Catherine. 2000. *The Visible Human Project: Informatic Bodies and Posthuman Medicine.* New York: Routledge.

Wallis, Claudia, and Kristina Dell. 2004. "What Makes Teens Tick." *Time* (May 10): 56–59.

Warner, Michael. 1991. "Introduction: Fear of a Queer Planet." *Social Text* 29: 3–17.

Wehrli, F. 1992. "The Origins and Future of Nuclear Magnetic Resonance Imaging." *Physics Today* 45:34–42.

Weiss, Rick. 1994. "Back Pain and MRIs: Vivid Images Are a Mixed Blessing." *Washington Post* (July 19): Z7.

Weiten, Wayne. 2003. *Psychology: Themes and Variations.* 6th ed. Belmont, CA: Wadsworth.

Westbrook, Catherine, and Carolyn Kaut. 1993. *MRI in Practice.* Boston: Blackwell Scientific.

Wilgus, Beverly, and Jack Wilgus. 2006. "The Magic Mirror of Life: An Appreciation of the Camera Obsura." Retreived May 25, 2006 (http://brightbytes.com/cosite/cohome.html).

Williams, Hywel, and Andres Pembroke. 1989. "Sniffer Dogs in the Melanoma Clinic?" *Lancet* 1:734.

Willis, Carolyn, Susannah Church, Claire Guest, W. Andrew Cook, Noel McCarthy, Anthea Bransbury, Martin Church, and John Church. 2004. "Olfactory Detection of Human Bladder Cancer By Dogs: Proof of Principle Study." *British Medical Journal* 329(7468): 712–715.

Willis, Deborah. 2005. *Family, History, Memory: Recording African-American Life.* New York: Hylas Publishing.

Wobarst, Anthony. 1999. *Looking Within: How X-ray, CT, MRI, Ultrasound, and Other Medical Images Are Created and How They Help Save Lives.* Berkeley: University of California Press.

Wolski, C.A. 2006. "In Contrast." *Medical Imaging Magazine.* Retrieved October 15, 2006 (http://www.medicalimagingmag.com/issues/articles/2006-05_02.asp).

World Health Organization [WHO]. 2000. *The World Health Report 2000: Health Systems: Improving Performance.* Geneva: Switzerland: Office of Publications.

——. 2006. *The World Health Report 2006: Working Together for Health.* Geneva: Switzerland: Office of Publications.

Yoxen, Edward. 1987. "Seeing with Sound: A Study of the Development of Medical Images." In *The Social Construction of Technological Systems: New Directions in the Sociology and History of Technology,* edited by W. Bijker, T. Hughes, and T. Pinch, 281–372. Cambridge, MA: MIT Press.

Yu, Jeong-Sik, Sang-Wook Yoon, Mi-Suk Park, Jei Hee Lee, and Ki Whang Kim. 2005. "Eosinophilic Hepatic Necrosis: Magnetic Resonance Imaging and Computed Tomography Comparison." *Journal of Computed Assisted Tomography* 29(6): 765–771.

Zinn, Howard. 1995. *A People's History of the United States, 1492–Present.* New York: HarperCollins.

Zola, Irving. 1972. "Medicine as an Institution of Social Control." *American Sociological Review* 20:487–504.

Index